# PREFACE

This Pocket Guide is based on the textbook *EMT Prehospital Care* by Mark Henry, MD, and Ed Stapleton, EMT-P, (W.B. Saunders Company, 1992). It is intended to provide the EMT with guidelines and helpful hints to review on the way to a run and documentation aids to refer to at the receiving hospital. Regardless of whatever text the EMT is familiar with, this guide reflects current treatment recommendations for specific basic life support prehospital skills that are consistent with current medical standards. Its pocket size is designed for ready access and can be carried conveniently in a uniform pocket or in a response vehicle's glove compartment.

Emergency medical service (EMS) is a relatively new and dynamic field that is rapidly evolving. These treatment protocols should not be considered the final word; they need to be constantly updated to reflect current standards of care.

## Acknowledgments

This book would not have been possible without the diligence, patience, and cooperation of the following: Margaret Biblis; Captain Forrest Dalton, EMT; Matthew Gorgen; Mark Henry, MD; Ed Stapleton, EMT-P; Dave Prout; the New York State Depart-

ment of Health, EMS Program; the New York City Emergency Medical Services; and the Omaha Fire Department, EMS Bureau.

## Important Note

The protocols included in this pocket guide are from the New York State EMS Program, the New York City Emergency Medical Services, and the Omaha Fire Department's EMS Service Program. Although these protocols were derived by practicing experts in emergency care and are based in large part on national standards and guidelines, the reader must recognize that there are constant changes and variations from region to region. Therefore, the reader needs to become familiar with his or her local protocols and follow them scrupulously in the delivery of patient care whenever appropriate.

The figures and many of the tables, procedures, and treatment lists are taken from *EMT Prehospital Care* by Mark Henry, MD, and Ed Stapleton, EMT-P, (W.B. Saunders Company, 1992).

**W.B. SAUNDERS COMPANY**

*A Division of Harcourt Brace & Company*

The Curtis Center
Independence Square West
Philadelphia, PA 19106

**Library of Congress
Cataloging-in-Publication Data**

Dalton, Alice Twink.
Pocket guide for EMT prehospital care / Alice Twink Dalton, Mark C. Henry, Edward R. Stapleton.
p. cm.
ISBN 0–7216–3781–7
1. Emergency medicine—Handbooks, manuals, etc. 2. Emergency medical technicians—Handbooks, manuals, etc. I. Dalton, Alice Twink. II. Henry, Mark C. III. Stapleton, Edward R. IV. Title. [DNLM: 1. Emergencies—handbooks. 2. Emergency Medical Services—handbooks. 3. Emergency Medical Technicians—handbooks. WX 39 D152p 1994]
RC86.8.D35 1994
616.02′5—dc20
DNLM/DLC 93-23587

Pocket Guide for EMT Prehospital Care
ISBN 0–7216–3781–7



Printed in United States of America

Last digit is the print number: 9 8 7 6 5 4 3 2 1

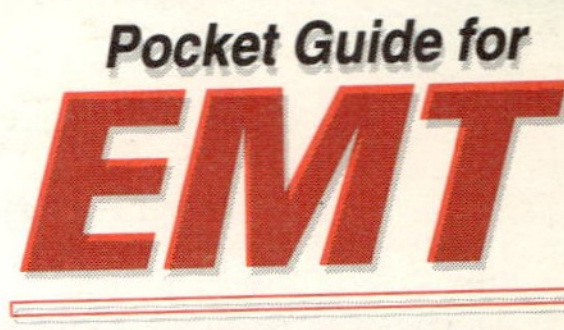


# PREHOSPITAL CARE

***Alice ("Twink") Dalton,*** ***RN, BSN, NRPM***
Instructor
Prehospital Education Program
Creighton University
Omaha, Nebraska

***Mark Henry, MD***
Associate Professor and Chairman
Department of Emergency Medicine
School of Medicine
State University of New York at Stony Brook
Stony Brook, New York

***Edward Stapleton, EMT-P***
Director of Prehospital Care and Education
University Hospital Instructor
Department of Emergency Medicine
School of Medicine
State University of New York at Stony Brook
Stony Brook, New York

**W.B. SAUNDERS COMPANY**
*A Division of Harcourt Brace & Company*
Philadelphia London Toronto Montreal Sydney Tokyo

# CONTENTS

# SCENE SURVEY

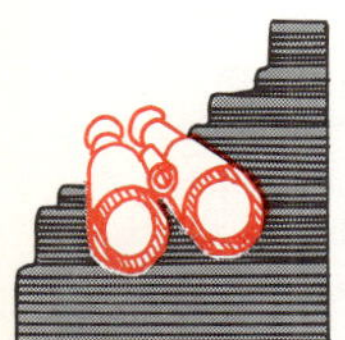

## "PLAIN-LABEL" CALLS

Emergency medical technicians (EMTs) frequently respond to calls such as "sick party," "man down," or "check a party" before complete or accurate medical information is known. To ensure that you are not caught off-guard

- Always carry the basic equipment for airway management and trauma.
- Don't hesitate to call in law enforcement if you sense a potentially hostile or dangerous situation.

## HAZARDS AT THE SCENE

As soon as an EMT arrives on the scene, he or she must quickly identify any hazards and determine the need for additional units. Before rushing into a scene, take 10 seconds to do a quick scene survey to ensure your own and others' safety. Dogs, downed power lines, hostile situations, and traffic hazards are common problems that will be discussed.

## Dogs

- When approaching a fenced yard, look for worn paths, bowls on the porch, and chains near the door.
- If a dog does not seem threatening, ignoring it may be the best choice. Dogs can sense fear, however, which may cause them to become more aggressive.
- If possible, ask a family member to control the dog.
- Depending on the seriousness of the situation, consider calling an animal control officer or the humane society before entering the scene. If access to the patient cannot be delayed, using a fire hose, fire extinguisher, or Mace may be necessary.
- If a pet is encountered after entering the scene, routine treatment may be perceived by the owner's dog as an attack. Confine the pet in a separate room, if possible, with all entrances and exits secured.
- Call law enforcement for help with a vicious attack dog, such as a pit bull.

## Downed Power Lines

- Any downed power line must be assumed to be hot.
- Follow your agency's protocols, but realize that access to a patient may be delayed until the power company gives the okay to proceed.

## Hostile Situations

- Follow your agency's policies for accessing law enforcement officers.
- Requests for police backup are made to a central communication center and occur when responding personnel or the patient is in a hostile situation. In some areas, "Expedite law enforcement" is the request made when a hostile situation is perceived. Law enforcement is dispatched as available. "Help a Firefighter/EMT" is made when responders are under attack. In this case, the closest police officers stop any activity and respond with lights and sirens.
- Trust your instincts. If the situation feels wrong, it probably is. Wait until police declare the area as being under control before entering.
- Do not allow your exit route to be blocked by bystanders. In some cases you must remove the patient and leave the area before treatment is started or completed.
- Do not enter a scene if weapons may be present (e.g., after shots have been fired or if a stabbing has occurred) until police indicate the area is under control. However, if you have already entered, weapons should be removed from the access of the patient or bystanders.

## Preserving Evidence

When weapons are present, care must be taken to ensure that firearms do not discharge and to preserve evidence as much as possible. If there are any signs of life, appropriate patient care must be delivered as soon as possible. Sometimes preservation of evidence may seem to interfere with good patient care. The following points may be helpful.

- If ropes are involved (as with a hanging victim), leave all knots intact. To cut someone down, cut the cord between the apparatus and the patient. To free the cord around the neck, arms, or legs, cut opposite the knot or two to three inches away.
- Leave openings made by a weapon in clothing intact. If clothing must be cut, cut away from the wound site. Collect all clothing and give to police at the hospital.
- If the victim is obviously dead, limit the number of people at the scene and limit movement of the body. Check for lividity and blood pooling on exposed body parts first; if present, further movement of the body is unnecessary. Seal the area until police arrive.
- If a weapon must be removed to ensure scene safety or to provide access to the patients, mark its position at both ends with chalk, a catheter, or pen, then tell responding police officers what you have done.
- Avoid grabbing the end of a rifle barrel; gun powder or blood that has blown back on the barrel is evidence. Instead, grab the barrel immediately above the wooden stock while placing your other hand on the butt plate to control where the rifle is pointed.
- Never point the barrel of a weapon at anyone. Always point weapons down toward the ground.
- You also may grab the knurl (carving on the stock) because prints can seldom be lifted from this part.
- Handguns can be picked up by using a pencil or

scissors in the finger guard or by grabbing the area immediately above the handle.

- Any automatic weapon after being fired is ready to fire again. A hammer that is pulled back is ready to fire again; if dropped, they can easily discharge.

### Traffic Hazards

- Most EMT deaths occur from traffic accidents—whether responding to a call, working at the scene, or transporting a patient to the hospital.
- Law enforcement should always be requested to control traffic at an accident scene.
- Always practice defensive driving; remember you are asking other drivers to yield the right of way, especially at intersections. Even if they are aware of your lights and sirens, they don't always yield.
- Inclement weather increases the risk of accidents; driving adjustments must be made for rain, sleet, and snow.

## EXTRICATION

The first responders survey the scene. Their primary concern is scene safety. Safe access must be ensured before patient care can be delivered. However, since access to the patient may occur before the patient can be removed, airway management, control of bleeding, and other procedures may be started before extrication.

Use the rapid extrication technique for any patient who shows signs of ventilatory failure, respiratory difficulty, or profound shock to institute life-saving measures.

Remember that the people involved in extrication are not the ones involved in patient care, except if there is a lack of personnel. In such cases, police officers, bystanders, and others may be able to assist.

## HAZARDOUS MATERIALS (HAZ-MAT)

A hazardous material action guide is given below. Identification of a HAZ-MAT scene can be difficult, especially since labeling of hazardous materials is required only for shipments of 1,000 pounds or more. Any time a vehicle is found to be carrying metal containers (marked or unmarked), barrels, or packages with directional markings or of unusual size or shape, suspect hazardous materials. Domestic labeling of hazardous materials can be found in the U.S. Department of Transportation's *Emergency Response Guidebook for Initial Response to Hazardous Materials Incidents*.

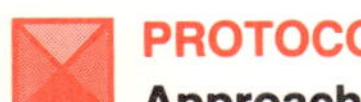

# PROTOCOL
## Approach to the Patient Exposed to a Hazardous Material

### Hazardous Material Action Guide*

All personnel regardless of training should follow the guidelines listed in regard to calls involving a hazardous material spill/incident:

1. **Always do a 10-second scene survey!**
2. Never underestimate the size of a spill or incident.
3. Establish and maintain proper communications with the borough or citywide dispatcher.
4. Stay upwind and upgrade at all times. Monitor weather and wind changes.
5. Do not breathe any smoke, fumes, or vapors.
6. Do not touch or walk through any spilled materials. You will only increase the size of the incident.
7. Do not eat, drink, or smoke at the scene of the incident. These are all direct routes of entry into the body.
8. Do not touch your face, nose, mouth, or eyes.
9. Eliminate all sources of ignition such as

*Continued.*

*From New York City Emergency Medical Services Basic Life Support Protocols, 1990.

flares, flames, sparks, smoking, flashes, flashlights, gas and diesel engines, and portable radios.

10 If your unit is the first on the scene, notify the dispatcher and give a condition in progress report. Request the assistance of the EPA, DEP, police and fire departments, and the EMS HAZ-MAT response team.

11 Do not drive through any spilled materials. You will only increase the size of the incident.

12 Identify the substance, if possible, using the *DOT Emergency Response Guidebook*. Inform the dispatcher of your findings.

13 Observe all safety precautions and directions as set forth by the incident commander, police and fire departments, EPA, DEP.

14 **All orders should be taken face to face!**

15 Remain clear of all restricted areas until declared safe by the incident commander.

## Procedure for Decontaminating Victims of a Haz-Mat Incident

1 Take the victim to a safe area where all clothing can be removed and an initial washdown can take place.

NOTE: *This should not be the staging area where patient care is taking place.* This area should be warm enough so that patients do not become hypothermic. Once clothing is removed it needs to be placed away from the decontamination area. Run-off from the washdown should flow away from all personnel.

2 Washdown of exposed areas must be done for a minimum of 10 to 15 minutes if the use of water or a water solution is the approach of choice.

NOTE: *Remember that some hazardous materials should not be washed away with water.* Once the type of material to which the patient has been exposed is identified, a determination can be made from experts (medical control; federal, state, local health or environment experts; or CHEMTREC) on the amount of time required for a washdown.

NOTE: Make sure that the run-off from the decontamination will not endanger other rescue personnel or other safe areas.

NOTE: Rescue personnel should make sure that they do not become contaminated during the decontamination process. Protective clothing and self-contained breathing apparatus might be necessary for certain types of hazardous materials.

3 Move the victim to another area for a second washdown or definitive patient care.

4 Decontaminate any vehicle that has been exposed to any hazardous material before it is used again.

*Continued.*

5 Place all contaminated clothing removed from victims and rescuers in an appropriate container that is sealed and sent to an approved area.

NOTE: The agency responsible for containment should be able to provide guidance on how to dispose of these items.

**Rescuers are apt to become contaminated. If this occurs, full decontamination procedures are to be followed for the rescuer before moving to the area for patient care.** ■

Common toxic gas exposure may be missed. Suspect, for example, carbon monoxide poisoning if all members of a household are ill, especially during the winter. To differentiate between food poisoning and a toxic gas, ask if the family has a pet. If the pet is sick or has died (birds are especially sensitive), the possibility of a toxic gas is high.

General signs and symptoms of toxic gas exposure include headache, drowsiness, fatigue, loss of appetite, nausea, and vomiting. These all are common in people painting or varnishing in an enclosed space, parking garage attendants, and firefighters after a fire. Treatment for toxic gases are listed in Table 1–1.

If an accident has resulted in a gasoline leak or if hazardous materials have been spilled, the risk of ignition must be considered.

**TABLE 1–1 ■ Toxic Gases**

| Gas | Properties | Physiologic Effect | Treatment |
|---|---|---|---|
| **SIMPLE ASPHYXIANTS** | | | |
| Carbon dioxide ($CO_2$) | Odorless, colorless | Simple asphyxiant; concentrations of 10% in atmosphere → unconsciousness | $O_2$ |
| Methane ($CH_4$) | Odorless, colorless | Simple asphyxiant | $O_2$ |
| **CHEMICAL ASPHYXIANTS** | | | |
| Carbon monoxide (CO) | Odorless, colorless | Asphyxiation (COHb) | $O_2$ |
| Cyanide (CN) | Bitter almonds, pink | Chemical asphyxiant, cyanide | Lilly Cyanide Kit |

*Continued on following page*

**TABLE 1–1 ■ Toxic Gases *Continued***

| Gas | Properties | Physiologic Effect | Treatment |
|---|---|---|---|
| **CHEMICAL ASPHYXIANTS** *Continued* | | | |
| Hydrogen sulfide ($H_2S$) | Powerful nauseating smell (olfactory fatigue), colorless | Chemical asphyxiant like CN with irritant properties | Lilly Cyanide Kit |
| **IRRITANT GASES (IRRITATION PROPORTIONAL TO SOLUBILITY)** | | | |
| Sulfur dioxide ($SO_2$) | Rotten eggs, colorless | Intensely irritating to eyes, nose, throat; usually upper airway effects | Supportive |
| Ammonia ($NH_3$) | Noxious, colorless | Intensely irritating to eyes, nose, throat; usually upper airway effects | Supportive |

| Gas | Properties | Physiologic Effect | Treatment |
|---|---|---|---|
| Hydrogen chloride (HCl) | Chlorine, colorless, or white mist | Irritant; delayed effects reported; myocardial irritability in PVC exposure reported; may be secondary to CO | Supportive |
| Chlorine ($Cl_2$) | Chlorine, greenish yellow | Irritant; pulmonary edema | Supportive |
| **IRRITANTS (LESS SOLUBLE THAN ABOVE)** | | | |
| Phosgene ($COCl_2$) | Mowed hay, colorless | Irritant; poorly perceived in concentrations capable of producing toxic effects; pulmonary edema after latent period | Supportive |
| Nitogen dioxides ($NO_2$, $N_2$, $O_4$) | Pungent odor, reddish brown | Only mild irritant to eye and respiratory tract; pulmonary edema; bronchiolitis | Supportive steroids might be considered |

*Continued on following page*

TABLE 1–1 ■ Toxic Gases *Continued*

| Gas | Properties | Physiologic Effect | Treatment |
|---|---|---|---|
| **NONIRRITANT (NOTE SPECIFIC PATHOLOGIC EFFECT)** | | | |
| Arsine ($AsH_3$) | Garlic, colorless | Nonirritating; attaches to sulfhydryl groups of Hb; hemolysis, acute renal failure, jaundice | $O_2$, transfusion since arsine nondialyzable, and dialysis for acute renal failure |

- Do not allow bystanders near the area to smoke, even if they must be removed by police.
- Motor vehicles involved in an accident should be shut off. If necessary, battery cables should be cut or unfastened.
- Response vehicles should be parked at a safe distance so their engines cannot ignite flammable material in the area.
- Leaking fuel needs to be removed according to HAZ-MAT standards (see page 7).

For radiation accidents, call Radiation Emergency Assistance Center/Training Site (REACT/TS) at (615)576-3131 Monday through Friday 8:00 A.M. to 4:30 P.M. At other times, call the Oak Ridge Hospital (Kentucky) at (615)481-1000, beeper 241.

For a HAZ-MAT accident (including radioactive materials), call Chemtrex at 800-424-9300 (24-hour service).

## INFECTION CONTROL

Table 1–2 gives infection control guidelines for prehospital care services.

**TABLE 1–2 ■ New York State Department of Health Infection Control Guidelines for Prehospital Care Services**

| Infection | Mode of Transmission | Recommended Precautions | Relative Risk in EMT Setting |
|---|---|---|---|
| AIDS/HIV (human immunodeficiency virus) | Needlestick, blood splash into mucous membranes (e.g., eyes, mouth), or blood contact of open wound | Universal precautions. | Low—no cases reported (Risk among health care workers in general is very low) |
| Chicken pox | Respiratory secretions and contact with moist vesicles | Gloves and hand washing. | None if immune. Significant if not immune |

| Infection | Mode of Transmission | Recommended Precautions | Relative Risk in EMT Setting |
|---|---|---|---|
| Common cold | Contact with respiratory secretions | Hand washing. Avoid contact of infectious materials with eyes, nose, or mouth. | Unknown—probably significant if in early stages |
| Diarrhea<br>*Campylobacter*<br>*Cryptosporidium*<br>*Giardia*<br>*Salmonella*<br>*Shigella*<br>Viral<br>*Yersinia* | Fecal/oral | Gloves for direct contact with stool (feces) and hand washing. | Unknown—probably low, providing hands are washed after contact with stool |

*Continued on following page*

**TABLE 1–2 ■ New York State Department of Health Infection Control Guidelines for Prehospital Care Services *Continued***

| Infection | Mode of Transmission | Recommended Precautions | Relative Risk in EMT Setting |
|---|---|---|---|
| Epiglottitis due to *Haemophilus influenzae* (usually seen in very young children) | Contact with respiratory secretions | Masks. | Unknown—probably low |
| German measles (rubella) | Respiratory droplets and contact with respiratory secretions | Masks. | Unknown—susceptible persons are at increased risk |
| Hepatitis A | Fecal/oral | Gloves and hand washing. | Minimal |

| Infection | Mode of Transmission | Recommended Precautions | Relative Risk in EMT Setting |
|---|---|---|---|
| Hepatitis B | Needlestick, blood splash into mucous membranes (e.g., eye or mouth), or blood contact of open wound. Possible exposure during mouth-to-mouth resuscitation | Universal precautions. | Significant (6–30% chance) if exposed to blood of a hepatitis B carrier and no pre- or postexposure prophylaxis is provided |
| Hepatitis C | As with hepatitis B | As with hepatitis B. | Unknown—probably low |

*Continued on following page*

**TABLE 1–2 ■ New York State Department of Health Infection Control Guidelines for Prehospital Care Services *Continued***

| Infection | Mode of Transmission | Recommended Precautions | Relative Risk in EMT Setting |
|---|---|---|---|
| Herpes simplex (cold sores) | Contact of mucous membrane with moist lesions. Fingers are at particular risk for becoming infected | Gloves. | Unknown—probably significant if lesions are present (most people have antibodies) |
| Herpes zoster (shingles) localized, disseminated (see chickenpox) | Contact with moist lesions | Gloves and hand washing. | Localized—very low and only if a person has not had chicken pox |

| Infection | Mode of Transmission | Recommended Precautions | Relative Risk in EMT Setting |
|---|---|---|---|
| Influenza | Airborne | Masks. | Unknown—probably significant during flu epidemics |
| Legionnaires' disease | No person-to-person transmission | None | None |
| Lice: head, body, pubic | Close head-to-head contact. Both body and pubic lice require intimate contact (usually sexual) or sharing of intimate clothing | Gloves and hand washing. | Unknown—head may be significant. Body and pubic probably not a risk |

*Continued on following page*

**TABLE 1–2 ■ New York State Department of Health Infection Control Guidelines for Prehospital Care Services *Continued***

| Infection | Mode of Transmission | Recommended Precautions | Relative Risk in EMT Setting |
|---|---|---|---|
| Measles | Respiratory droplets and contact with nasal or throat secretions. Highly communicable | Masks. | Unknown—probably significant if lesions are present (most people have antibodies) |
| Meningitis | | | |
| *Meningococcus* | Contact with respiratory secretions | Masks. | Unknown—probably low unless mouth-to-mouth ventilation is done |

| Infection | Mode of Transmission | Recommended Precautions | Relative Risk in EMT Setting |
|---|---|---|---|
| Meningitis *Cont'd* | | | |
| *Haemophilus influenzae* (usually seen in very young children) | Contact with respiratory secretions | Masks. | Unknown—probably low |
| Viral | Fecal/oral | Hand washing. | Unknown—probably low |
| Mumps (infectious parotitis) | Respiratory droplets and contact with saliva | Masks. | Unknown—most adults are immune |
| Scabies | Close body contact | Wash hands and arms carefully after contact | Unknown—probably low |

*Continued on following page*

**TABLE 1–2 ■ New York State Department of Health Infection Control Guidelines for Prehospital Care Services *Continued***

| Infection | Mode of Transmission | Recommended Precautions | Relative Risk in EMT Setting |
|---|---|---|---|
| Tuberculosis, pulmonary | Airborne | Mask on patient. | Unknown—depends on level of patient's infectivity and contact time. Most transmission occurs in household setting where duration of exposure is extended |

| Infection | Mode of Transmission | Recommended Precautions | Relative Risk in EMT Setting |
| --- | --- | --- | --- |
| Wounds, infected and draining | Contact—more of a concern for cross-contamination | Gloves and hand washing. | Probably none |

Modified from A Prehospital Care Provider's Guide to AIDS. Albany: New York State Department of Health, January 1990.

## PROTOCOL
## Patients with Communicable Disease

### Control of Infection

All health care providers are responsible for limiting the possibility of cross-infection among patients and personnel. The following precautions are to be followed at *all* times:

1 Wash hands thoroughly after any patient contact.
2 Do not use linen or disposable items on more than one patient.
3 Linens and items that are not designed for multiple use are to be appropriately disposed of as soon as possible.
4 All equipment should be maintained in a clean and sanitary condition.

### Handling Patients with Possible Communicable Disease

#### *During the Call*

1 Assess and treat the patient according to standard protocols.
2 Wash hands and forearms thoroughly after contact with the patient.
3 Wear appropriate protective gear according to four categories:
   a **Category I—Blood / Body Fluid Precautions**
   *Gloves only:* With the high incidence of viral disease in our patient population, all

blood/body fluids must be presumed to be infectious. Therefore, EMTs should wear nonsterile, disposable gloves whenever they may contact blood/body fluids such as feces, urine, or skin infections.

b **Category II—Respiratory Precautions**
*Mask only:* Tuberculosis is on the rise, especially among the indigent and alcoholics, and may be spread by close contact with respiratory secretions. EMTs should place a mask on any patient with a cough that has lasted more than 48 hours.

c **Category III—Secretion Precautions**
*Mask and gloves:* Such diseases as varicella (chicken pox), rubella (German measles), rubeola (measles), and meningococcal meningitis may be spread by close contact with respiratory secretions and/or skin rashes. As a general rule, EMTs should use gloves and mask if a patient has a skin rash and fever.

d **Category IV—Contamination Precautions**
*Gloves, mask, and gown:* These precautions should be taken when an EMT identifies a patient who is grossly contaminated with infectious material, which would otherwise contaminate the EMT's uniform or when there is a chance of splattering body fluids.

*Continued.*

4 Avoid direct contact with body fluids and secretions, including sputum, blood, urine, and feces.
5 Note all personnel in contact with the patient.

*At the Receiving Facility*

1 Report appropriate information to the emergency department staff.
2 Request that the facility notify the EMS office as soon as a positive diagnosis is made.

*After the Call*

1 Report incident to the supervisor on duty.
2 Dispose of linens according to hospital protocols.
3 Thoroughly clean and disinfect all parts of the ambulance compartment that were in contact with the patient.
4 Change uniform if necessary.

**Recommendations for Decontamination and Cleaning of Rescue Vehicles***

*Clean-Up Kit*

- Household utility gloves
- Plastic spray bottle with cleaning agent
- Plastic spray bottle with disinfectant solution or bottle with concentrated household bleach to be diluted with water (1:100 dilution approximates ¼ cup bleach per gallon of water)

*From A Prehospital Care Provider's Guide to AIDS. Albany: New York State Department of Health, January 1990.

- Disposable toweling
- Plastic bags (hospital red bags and household plastic bags)
- Basket or carrier to hold cleaning supplies.

***Clean-Up Procedure after Each Call***

1 Prepare vehicle for cleaning and decontamination:

  **a** Always wear utility gloves throughout entire clean-up procedure.

  **b** Remove used or soiled linen and place in designated bag for laundering. Either leave laundry at the hospital or reprocess in the EMS laundry using warm water, detergent, and bleach, as recommended on the product labels.

  **c** Discard any soiled dressings, bloody materials, and other contaminated, non-sharps waste in a red bag and leave at the hospital.

  **d** Place reusable equipment that needs reprocessing in plastic bag (any color other than red).

  **e** Check the vehicle for any needles or other sharps that may have been left and carefully dispose in a sharps container.

2 Check for areas soiled with blood and other visible body substances and remove.

  **a** Remove moist blood and other body sub-

*Continued.*

stances with paper toweling and discard in a red bag.

- **b** Spray cleaner on affected area and remove any remaining blood or body substance. Dispose of towels in red bag.
- **c** Spray disinfectant on affected area, wipe over the surface, and allow to air-dry. Dispose of towels in red bag.

**3** Use spray cleaner on remaining surfaces with which the patient had contact as well as surfaces that were used in the course of providing prehospital care. Wipe the surface with toweling and allow to air-dry.

### *Periodic Cleaning of Rescue Vehicles*

On a regular basis (e.g., weekly or monthly), as determined by the frequency of vehicle use and obvious need, the floors, walls, interior and exterior of cabinets and drawers, benches, and other surfaces, should be thoroughly cleaned. The same cleaning agent used between cases can be used for this more extensive cleaning. A supply kit should be kept in a central location for this purpose (e.g., pail, reusable cleaning cloths that are laundered after use, and a supply of cleaning agents). Wipe with toweling and allow to air-dry.

NOTE: Bleach solution should be made up fresh at the time of use or daily.

Since carpeting and permeable seat covers in the patient compartment of ambulances are more difficult to clean than nonpermeable surfaces, their use is not recommended. ■

## RADIO REPORTS AND CODES

It is important for hospitals to be notified of the arrival of seriously ill or injured patients. All of the following information should be relayed to the hospital.

### Hospital Radio Reports

1. Identify responding department and unit number.
2. Give patient information. (If there is more than one, designate them as Patient 1, Patient 2, etc.)
   - Age and sex
   - Chief complaint and/or mechanism of injury
   - Level of consciousness and vital signs
   - Significant symptoms and assessment findings
   - Enough pertinent history to clarify the problem (preexisting medical conditions, allergies, medications, etc.).

NOTE: *Outstanding assessment findings may take precedence and need to be reported first* (e.g., "Adult male, age 50, found pulseless, apneic, and unresponsive; CPR in progress").

3. Describe treatment given (e.g., "oxygen per na-

sal cannula at 4 liters," or "traction splint applied") and patient's response.

4. Give estimated time of arrival (ETA). Notify hospital of any delay in transport or unusual circumstances.
5. When interfacing with advanced life support (ALS), give short reports to incoming paramedics (e.g., chief complaint or mechanism of injury, vital signs, and initial treatment) because patient status may be very different from dispatch and continuity of care depends on it.
6. On arrival at the emergency department, submit a verbal report summarizing this information to responsible medical personnel. Submit the hospital copy of the Ambulance Call Report to the responsible emergency department personnel after crew members have had the opportunity to review it.

NOTE: Because radio reports can be monitored by anyone with a police-band radio, use discretion when broadcasting.

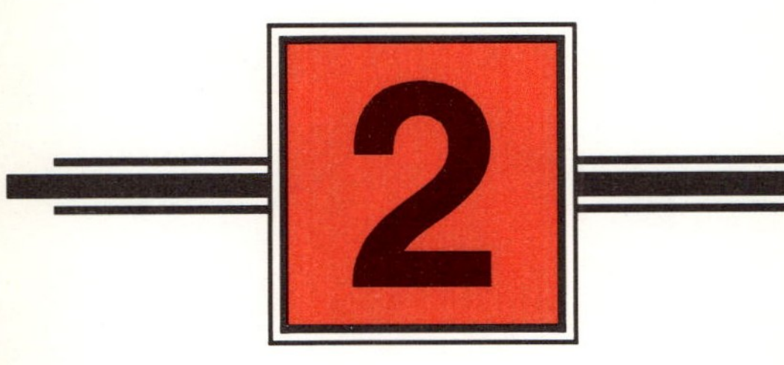

# PATIENT SURVEY

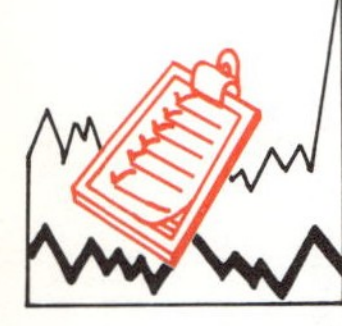

After the scene survey is complete, the EMT does a patient survey. The patient survey is to determine a working diagnosis from which treatment, transportation, and triage decisions are all dependent. The patient survey consists of two parts: the physical examination and history-taking.

## MECHANISM OF INJURY

Recognizing the mechanism(s) of injury (MOI) helps determine the sites and seriousness of the patient's condition (Table 2–1). This fact also must be relayed to the hospital staff for the same reason. Keep in mind that a patient who has suffered a significant MOI may initially present as being stable with relatively normal vital signs, but depending on the MOI and kinetics involved, his or her status may subsequently rapidly deteriorate from an internal

**TABLE 2–1 ■ Mechanisms of Injury and Associated Injuries**

| Mechanism | Common Associated Injuries |
|---|---|
| Head-on collisions | Head and spinal trauma |
| | Chest and abdominal trauma |
| | Flail chest |
| | Pneumothorax |
| | Internal hemorrhage |
| | Lower extremity trauma |
| | Knee, femur, hip |
| | Upper extremity trauma |
| | Protection injury |
| Side collision | Head and spinal trauma |
| | Chest and abdominal trauma |
| | Lateral chest wall injury |
| | Flail chest |
| | Pneumothorax |
| | Internal hemorrhage |

| Mechanism | Common Associated Injuries |
|---|---|
| Side collision *Cont'd* | Upper extremity trauma |
| | Shoulder, clavicle, humerus |
| | Lower extremity trauma |
| | Hip/acetabulum |
| Rear-end collision | Head and spinal trauma |
| | Contra coup |
| | Whiplash |
| Rotational collision force | Varies according to vector; person closest to impact point most injured |
| Falls | Types of injury depend on impact point |
| Feet first | Calcaneus (heel) |
| | Lower extremity |
| | Spine |
| Outstretched arm | Wrist, elbow, humerus, shoulder |
| Penetrating knife injuries | Type of injury depends on size, direction and location |
| Missile injuries | Type of injury depends on velocity, location, and range |

injury. Thus, a patient with normal signs and symptoms plus a significant MOI warrants rapid transport and frequent assessments (at least every 10 to 15 minutes).

If cameras are used to document an MOI, close-up shots are necessary at night. Patient treatment or transport should never be delayed to take pictures.

## PHYSICAL EXAMINATION

The physical examination is divided into the primary and secondary assessments. The primary assessment includes treatment for actual or potential life-threatening situations and is based on a priority system that does not change. However, the assessment steps for a medical patient differs slightly from those for a trauma patient, as shown in Table 2–2. The secondary assessment includes vital signs, head-to-toe survey, and neurologic examination.

### Primary Assessment

The primary assessment procedure shown in the next section is used for both trauma and medical patients. When there is enough help, several assessment steps and treatment can be done simultaneously (e.g., applying direct pressure to a spurting artery while the level of consciousness is assessed and oxygen is administered).

#### *Special Considerations*

- A patient who is talking, or a child who is crying, has an open airway and is breathing.
- Adequate breathing for both medical and trauma

**TABLE 2–2 ■ Basic Assessment Steps for the Trauma and Medical Patient**

| Trauma | Medical |
|---|---|
| 1. Immobilize cervical spine | |
| **AIRWAY** | |
| 2. Establish responsiveness | 2. Establish responsiveness |
| 3. Ensure a clear airway | 3. Ensure a clear airway |
| **BREATHING** | |
| 4. Check for breathing | 4. Check for breathing |
| 5. Evaluate the adequacy of breathing | 5. Evaluate the adequacy of breathing |
| 6. Look for obvious chest wounds | 6. Look for retractions, accessory muscle use |
| **CIRCULATION** | |
| 7. Check for a pulse | 7. Check for a pulse |

*Continued on following page*

**TABLE 2–2 ■ Basic Assessment Steps for the Trauma and Medical Patient *Continued***

| Trauma | Medical |
|---|---|
| **CIRCULATION** *Continued* | |
| 8. Look for obvious external bleeding and open wounds | 8. Look for obvious s/s of internal bleeding |
| 9. Evaluate adequacy of circulation | 9. Evaluate adequacy of circulation |
| **DISABILITY** | |
| 10. Determine the level of consciousness | 10. Determine the level of consciousness |
| 11. Evaluate the neurologic (CNS) function | 11. Evaluate the neurologic (CNS) function |
| **EXPOSE** | |
| 12. Expose the head and trunk to identify signs of major trauma | 12. Expose the chest, trunk or legs as necessary to identify clues to major illness |

patients is evaluated by the ability to speak in complete sentences. Aggressive airway management with appropriate oxygen therapy is the single most important action care providers do to save lives (regardless of their level of training).

- Checking for chest wounds (e.g., bruising, open wounds, and flail segments) applies to both breathing and circulation. Chest wounds disrupt the adequacy of ventilation and have a tendency to bleed.
- Oxygen therapy is an essential part of treatment and is usually initiated during the primary assessment (see Oxygen Administration Protocol on page 50).

## Approach to a Prehospital Patient*

1. Initial scene assessment
   a. Assess the scene for safety.
   b. Note the number of patients, mechanisms of injury, environmental hazards, and other pertinent data.
   c. Call for additional personnel and equipment if needed.
2. Perform expanded primary assessment, and resuscitate if necessary.
   a. **Airway**
      (1) Is the airway open, and will it stay open?
      (2) Use the jaw-thrust without head-tilt for all patients with suspected spinal inju-

*Modified from Manual for Emergency Medical Technicians. Emergency Medical Services Program. Albany: New York State Department of Health, 1990.

ries. Manually stabilize the head and neck, even when cervical collars are used.

(3) Suction the patient's pharynx and insert oral/nasal airway, if necessary. Patients who have been drinking alcohol usually vomit. Place in coma position if no trauma.

b. **Breathing**

(1) Is breathing present, and is it adequate? Respirations below 12 or more than 30 per minute usually require mechanical assistance, such as a bag-valve-mask.

(2) Can the patient take a deep breath? Any pain during breathing? If the patient can speak in complete sentences, one can assume adequate respiration.

(3) Inspect, palpate, and auscultate the chest. Cover wounds with occlusive dressings. Stabilize flail segments. Snoring, gurgling, wheezing, and high-pitched sounds (stridor) suggest airway obstruction.

(4) Note skin color. Blue discoloration indicates poor oxygenation. Give high-concentration oxygen and, if needed, positive-pressure ventilation by bag-valve-mask.

c. **Circulation**

(1) Is a pulse present?

(2) Is obvious, serious internal/external bleeding present?

(3) Check nail bed refill. Delayed capillary refill indicates poor perfusion but may be normal in cold temperatures and some elderly patients. Capillary refill is

not an absolute sign when assessing for shock. A single sign or symptom rarely gives an accurate picture of the patient's condition.

(4) Pale, cool, sweaty, or cyanotic skin suggests poor perfusion and cardiovascular function. Sweating may not always be present or to the usual degree when patients are taking certain blood pressure or heart medications. Pallor and cyanosis begins around the mouth, nose, and ears.

(5) Use pulse to determine approximate blood pressure: If *radial pulse* is present = 80 mm Hg systolic; if *femoral pulse* is present = 70 mm Hg systolic; if *carotid pulse* is present = 60 mm Hg systolic.

(6) Is the patient in shock?

(7) Obtain baseline set of vital signs.

(8) Support circulation as necessary.

(9) Treat for shock.

(10) Elevate legs if fractures are not present.

(11) Use military antishock trousers (MAST), unless contraindicated.

d. **Disability:**

(1) Assess the patient's **level of consciousness** (LOC), which is the most sensitive indicator of central nervous system function. The mnemonic AVPU (alert, verbal, painful, or unresponsive) is useful for determining mental status.

(a) Alert: Adult patients know their

## TABLE 2–3 ■ Glasgow Coma Scale

| | | |
|---|---|---|
| **EYE OPENING** | | |
| Spontaneous | 4 | |
| To voice | 3 | |
| To pain | 2 | |
| None | 1 | |
| **VERBAL RESPONSE** | | |
| Oriented | 5 | |
| Confused | 4 | **Patient's Best Verbal Response:** Arouse patient with voice or painful stimulus. |
| Inappropriate words | 3 | |
| Incomprehensible sounds | 2 | |
| None | 1 | |
| **MOTOR RESPONSE** | | |
| Obeys command | 6 | **Patient's Best Motor Response:** Response to command or painful stimulus. |
| Localizes pain | 5 | |
| Withdraw (pain) | 4 | |

| **MOTOR RESPONSE** *Continued* | |
|---|---|
| Flexion (pain) | 3 |
| Extension (pain) | 2 |
| None | 1 |
| TOTAL GCS SCORE | 3-15 |

The Glasgow Coma Scale defines a patient's neurologic status. A patient with a total score of less than 8 usually requires hyperventilation. In some areas, the score determines to what hospital the patient will be taken.

From American College of Surgeons, Resources for Optimal Care of the Injured Patient, 1993.

name, where they are, and day of the week. For infants or children, see page 59.

(b) Verbal: Patient responds to verbal stimuli. Record response. See Glasgow Coma Scale (GCS) (Table 2–3).

(c) Painful: Patient responds only to pain.

(d) Unresponsive: Patient does not respond verbally or react to pain.

NOTE: AVPU determines what it takes to get a response; the GCS ranks the response by number.

(2) Assess the **pupils:** If patient has unequal pupils and altered LOC, hyperventilate at 24 to 30 times per minute.

(3) Perform quick assessment of ability to move extremities.

(4) Apply a rigid collar and stabilize the head and neck.

e. **Expose** portions of the patient's body as appropriate to locate life-threatening problems or indications of serious illness (e.g., rashes, red streaks, track marks, edema, and bruises). When weapons have been used (e.g., guns or knives), all clothing must be removed to determine all entrance and exit wounds.

3. **Immediate Transport Decision:** Vital signs, secondary survey and field treatment may be done at the scene *only* if the patient is stable!

4. **Vital Signs:** Obtain and record the following on every patient initially, and repeat as needed.

   a. Pulse—location, rate and quality.

   b. Respirations—rate and quality. ■

c. Blood pressure—systolic and diastolic. If you hear sounds all the way to "0," the last sound change heard is the diastolic. Then record as three numbers (e.g., 180/110/0).
d. Skin—color, temperature, and moisture.

5. **Secondary Survey:** Complete as indicated by the patient's condition.
   a. Reassure and inform the patient about assessment and treatment.
   b. Obtain and record chief complaint, subjective information, any pertinent history of present or past illness, and any pertinent medical information from the patient, family, and bystanders. Check for medical identification bracelet, necklace, or card in wallet.
6. **Field Treatment.** Administer appropriate treatment in order of priority. See Chapter 4, Chief Complaint or Injury, or Chapter 5, Trauma.

## Secondary Assessment

The secondary survey takes place after the primary survey has been completed and all potential life-threatening conditions have been managed. The scope of the secondary survey varies according to the patient problem and can be altered or modified by any life-threatening condition.

NOTE: In the acutely ill or injured patient, the EMT may never progress beyond the primary assessment.

A complete neurologic examination includes evaluating the level of consciousness by the Glas-

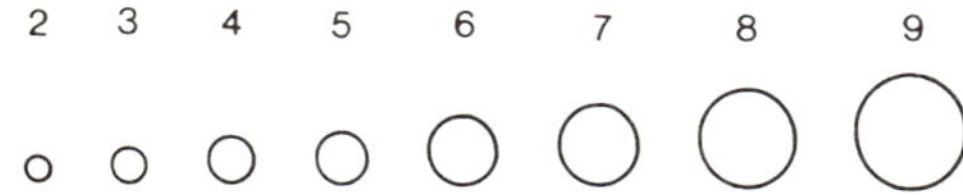


**Figure 2–1** This chart provides an accurate measurement of pupil diameter in millimeters.

gow Coma Scale (Table 2–3) and measuring pupil size and reaction time (Fig. 2–1).

Orientation refers to awareness of person, place, and time. The degree of orientation can be more specifically established by asking patients their name, the location, and the day or approximate time. Failure to answer all three questions correctly is called "disoriented times three" and is documented as such. If one of these components is missed, state exactly what was answered correctly (e.g., "Oriented to person and place" or "Oriented to person").

Confusion implies the patient is capable of some sustained conversation but gives incorrect answers or appears disoriented. If the patient becomes combative, recording exact patient behavior is much more useful than to state, "Patient is confused and combative."

## HISTORY-TAKING

History-taking is often the most significant part of patient assessment. Most medical and many trauma-related problems are diagnosed primarily on the basis of history. The components of history-taking include (1) chief complaint, (2) history of present illness, (3) past medical problems, (4) medications, and (5) allergies.

In general, the EMT should use open-ended questions but stay focused on the most important information. The patient is the best source for data; bystanders supplement but do not replace the patient's own history.

***Chief Complaint.*** The chief complaint is what the patient tells you is wrong or the reason the ambulance was called. Ask the patient, "What is bothering you the most right now?"

***History of Present Illness.*** Try to reconstruct the sequence of events by asking the following **general questions:**

- "When did the problem begin, and what were you doing when you first felt ill?"
- "How long have you felt ill? Has this happened before? What makes it better or worse?"
- "How many times has it occurred in the last hour (or since this morning, or since it started)?"
- "Do you have any other symptoms or problems?"
- "Have you done anything or taken any medicine for it?"

For **pain,** specific questions in addition to the general ones include:

- "How would you describe the pain? Can you point to it?"
- "Has the pain changed, or does it radiate anywhere?"
- "On a scale of one to ten, with ten being the worst, how would you rate it?"

For **dyspnea,** specific questions in addition to the general ones include:

- "Does activity make it better or worse?"
- "Has it happened before? What was wrong then? Is this like before?"
- "Are you allergic to anything?"
- "Have you recently had a cold, cough, or fever?" (This may indicate pneumonia or other infectious disease.)

For **headaches,** specific questions in addition to the general ones include:

- "Can you point to where it hurts the worst?"
- "How would you describe the pain? Has it changed?"
- "Does light affect it?"
- "Do you have any other symptoms or problems?"

For **nausea** and **vomiting,** specific questions in addition to the general ones include:

- "What did you eat before the episode? How long ago?"
- "What does the vomitus look like (e.g., coffee grounds)?"
- "How many times have you vomited?"
- "Can you keep water down?"

For **diarrhea,** specific questions in addition to the general ones include:

- "What does it look like (e.g., presence of mucus or blood)?"
- How many stools in the last 4 hours (or since onset)? (This is useful in determining the degree of dehydration that may be present.)

***Past Medical Problems.*** Past medical problems

are often related to the chief complaint. Be sure to ask the patient about the following conditions:

| ***Chief Complaint*** | ***Pertinent Data*** |
|---|---|
| Chest pain | Previous heart attack, angina, cardiac or lung problems |
| Dyspnea | Asthma, emphysema, chronic obstructive pulmonary disease (COPD), congestive heart failure (or "water in the lungs"), allergies, or exposure to chemicals |
| Headache | Stroke or high blood pressure |
| Nausea and vomiting | These nonspecific problems may be caused by anything from diabetes and ulcers to myocardial infarction, or food poisoning. History-taking is extremely important |
| Diarrhea | Ulcers or chronic gastrointestinal problems |
| Dizziness | Heart problems, ear infections, use of antibiotics or antihistamines, allergies, or blood pressure variances (either high or low) |

***Medications.*** Ask the patient about all prescriptions as well as all over-the-counter and recreational drugs.

- "What prescriptions are you taking?"
- "Do you take your medicine as directed, or do you sometimes skip a dose?"

- "Do you take drugs recreationally?"
  See also Poisoning and Drug Overdose, page 124.

***Allergies.*** Always ask the patient about any allergy. Depending on the situation, either specific drug reactions or insect and food allergies are more pertinent. See also Allergy/Anaphylaxis, page 93.

## PROTOCOL
## Oxygen Administration*

1 Assure that the patient's airway is open and that breathing and circulation are adequate. If not, perform obstructed airway maneuvers according to AHA/ARC standards.

2 If ventilations are present and adequate (>10/minute or <30/minute in an adult or >15/minute in a child) with normal skin color and clear lung sounds, **administer oxygen with a nasal cannula at 2–4 liters per minute (LPM).**

3 If ventilations are present and adequate with poor skin color and rales, rhonchi, or wheezes are present, **administer high flow oxygen with a mask-nonrebreather.**

  a Fill the bag to its capacity, then adjust the oxygen flow (usually 12 LPM) so the

*Modified from Manual for Emergency Medical Technicians. Emergency Medical Services Program. Albany: New York State Department of Health, 1990.

bag remains one-third full after an inspiration.

**Nasal cannula at 6 LPM is used only if a mask is not tolerated.**

4 If ventilations are present but inadequate (<10/minute or >30/minute in an adult or <15 in a child) and the patient is confused, restless, or cyanotic, administer 100 percent oxygen using a positive-pressure adjunctive device such as a **bag-valve-mask (BVM) with a reservoir.**

**A nonrebreathing mask is used only if a BVM is not tolerated.**

### Children

1 There is no contraindication for providing high-concentration oxygen for children in the prehospital setting.
2 Allow the parent to hold the face mask (about 6 to 8 inches from the child's face), which may be reassuring to the child.
3 Humidified oxygen is preferred, but dry oxygen is better than none.

### Patients with COPD

1 Oxygen should never be withheld from patients requiring it, even if they may already

*Continued.*

have a disabling condition such as chronic obstructive pulmonary disease.

2 Watch the patient carefully for any slowing of respirations. Be prepared to ventilate, if necessary.

3 If a patient who is already being maintained on oxygen therapy requires transport for a condition other than one requiring high-concentration oxygen, continue to administer oxygen at the previously prescribed rate of flow.

■

# SPECIAL PATIENTS

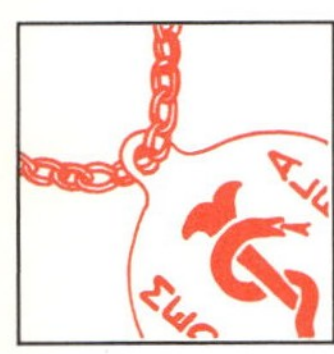

EMTs deal with a variety of patients who have special needs. Special problems in communication are

1. Elderly patients
   a. Treat with special respect
   b. Move patient with care
   c. Be sensitive to the spouse's concerns
   d. Bring dentures/glasses
   e. Keep warm, e.g., cover feet
   f. Lock doors, bring keys
   g. Arrange for care of pets
2. The sick or injured child
   a. Allow the parent to accompany the child
   b. Bring other objects that help make the child feel more secure
   c. Interact with both the parent and child
   d. Be honest with the child
3. Deaf patients
   a. When speaking to a person able to lip read, touch shoulder while looking directly at the

patient's face and speak in a normal tone of voice

   b. Use short, written questions, if necessary
   c. Be patient
   d. Explain what you are doing to the patient
4. Blind patients
   a. Maintain physical contact
   b. Describe in detail what you are doing
   c. If patient has a Seeing Eye dog, bring dog with the patient or arrange for care of the dog
5. Patients who speak another language
   a. Use a translator if patient either does not speak English or if the EMT is unsure of whether or not the patient understands questions
6. Confused patients
   a. Use simple terms
   b. Give simple explanations
   c. Reinforce orientation and simple explanations
   d. Allow patient ample time to respond
   e. Assume that the patient can understand what you say
7. Mentally retarded patients
   a. Give simple explanations and reinforcement
   b. Determine capability of patient to understand
   c. Distinguish mental from physical disability
   d. Assume that the patient can understand what you say

## PEDIATRICS

The awake but sick or injured child requires a different approach from that of an adult. Remember that normal respiratory and heart rates are faster in children. The only presenting sign of a severely ill infant may be that, in the parent's opinion, the child is "just not acting right."

### *Critical Pediatric Vital Signs**

1. Minimum ventilatory rates according to age groups:

| Age Group | If Respiratory Rate Is | Ventilate at (Minimum) |
|---|---|---|
| <2 yr | <15/min | 20/min |
| >2 yr | <10/min | 15/min |

2. Criteria for tachycardia:

| Age Group | Pulse Rate |
|---|---|
| <1 yr | >170/min |
| 1-6 yr | >150/min |
| >6 yr | >130/min |

3. Criteria for hypotension:

| Age Group | Systolic Blood Pressure |
|---|---|
| <2 yr | <60 mm Hg |
| >2 yr | <60 mm Hg |

*From Manual for Emergency Medical Technicians. Emergency Medical Services Program. Albany: New York State Department of Health, 1990.

4. Criteria for rapid respirations:

| *Age Group* | *Upper Limit* |
|---|---|
| <1 yr | 60/min |
| 1-5 yr | 40/min |
| >5 yr | 30/min |

5. Criteria for hypotension and indication for mast inflation in clinical shock:

| *Age Group* | *Systolic Blood Pressure* |
|---|---|
| <2 yr | <60 mm Hg |
| >2 yr | <70 mm Hg |

6. Approximate respiratory rate for hyperventilating child:

| *Age Group* | *Minimum Rate* |
|---|---|
| <2 yr | 30/min |
| >2 yr | 25/min |

Children are usually divided into five groups: infants (newborn to 1 year), toddlers (1 to 3 years), preschoolers (4 to 6 years), school-age children (6 to 11 years), and teenagers (11 to 19 years).

The approach to the pediatric patient is similar to that of adults (see page 39) but with the following special considerations.

### *Special Considerations*

- Assess and talk to the child at eye level.
- Listen to the **lung sounds** first since you do not know how long the child will remain quiet. If the child is old enough to understand, ask him or her to blow at your pen as if it were a candle. Listen on inhalation and exhalation.

- A strong cry is a good sign of a clear airway and good oxygen exchange.
- If the child has **stridor,** do not examine the oropharynx, except for direct visualization of a foreign body.
- Mottling of the trunk indicates inadequate perfusion. Suspect respiratory compromise or shock.
- Bulging fontanelles on an infant indicates increased intracranial pressure. Causes include infection (e.g., meningitis), subdural hematomas, or vigorous crying.
- Relatively small amounts of blood loss (e.g., 500 mL in a 50-lb. child) can cause shock.

## Approach to the Pediatric Patient*

1. Initial scene assessment
   a. Especially for toddlers and infants, a parent's presence may be a calming factor.
   b. Parents should be considered as patients also.
   c. Ask the parent to hold the child while you complete an assessment and deliver initial treatment, unless the parent's presence upsets the child.
2. Expanded primary assessment/resuscitation
   a. *Airway:* Identify and correct any existing or potential airway obstruction. If trauma is present, protect the cervical spine.
      (1) Insert oral or nasal airway as necessary. Nasal airways are not appropriate in infants or toddlers.

*Modified from New York State Basic Life Support Protocols and New York City EMS Academy training protocols.

(2) Hyperextension of the neck will occlude the airway of an infant or toddler.

b. *Breathing:* Identify and correct any existing or potentially compromising factors.
   (1) Presence of stridor, wheezing, and grunting (in infants) all indicate respiratory distress. Retractions (intercostal, suprasternal, and sternal) and see-saw respirations indicate severe respiratory distress.
   (2) How is the patient crying? A weak cry is more indicative of distress than a vigorous cry. Moaning is associated with shock.
   (3) Auscultate the chest before palpation. Equal lung sounds *do not* rule out pneumothorax because lung sounds echo from one side to the other.
   (4) Flail segments are rare.
   (5) Oxygen is best delivered to an infant using the blow-by technique, rather than having oxygen directly in an infant's face. Ventilate as necessary.

c. *Circulation:* Identify and correct any existing or potentially compromising factors.
   (1) Are peripheral *and* central pulses present? The pulse rate is a more accurate indicator of shock than any other vital sign.
   (2) Head wounds can be significant sources of blood loss in an infant or toddler.
   (3) Note the skin color and temperature on the extremities, especially the legs, and note where on the extremity the color and temperature change occurs.

d. *Disability:* If the child cannot move the extremities, apply a rigid collar (if appropriate size is available) or towel rolls, and stabilize the head and neck. If the child is in an infant seat or child restraint, immobilize as is. Consider the developmental age of the child, and assess the patient's pupils and level of consciousness as follows (see also Glasgow Coma Scale on page 224):
   (1) *Alert*—patient knows his or her name, where he or she is, and the day of the week. Toddler or infant recognizes parents.
   (2) *Verbal*—child is uninterested in events or dozing, but responds by turning head or stopping activity in response to sound.
   (3) *Painful*—child is hard to arouse but moans or moves when pinched.
   (4) *Unresponsive*—The child does not respond verbally or react to pain.

e. *Expose* the patient as appropriate to locate life-threatening problems. Look for rashes, red streaks, bruising, etc.

3. **Immediate transport decision:** *If the patient's condition warrants it, the vital signs, secondary survey, and treatment should be done en route to the hospital.*
4. Vital signs: Obtain and record the following information on every patient initially, and repeat as often as needed.
   a. *Pulse*—rate, location, and quality.
   b. *Respirations*—rate and quality and presence of retractions.

   c. *Blood pressure*—systolic and diastolic.
   d. *Skin*—color, temperature, and moisture.
4. Secondary survey: As for the adult patient, complete as indicated by the child's condition.
   a. For all infants and small children, perform a head-to-toe examination.
   b. Reassure and inform the child and parent about the treatment.
5. Field treatment: Administer appropriate treatment in order of priority. Refer to specific treatment protocols.
6. Notification: Notify the hospital of the arrival of a seriously ill or injured child.
   a. Patient information (same as for adult patients; see page 31).
   b. Notification of any delay in transport or unusual circumstances and estimated time of arrival (ETA).
7. Arrival at the hospital: At the emergency department submit a verbal report summarizing the above information and the written prehospital care report to the responsible medical personnel.

## Difficulty Breathing

### *History*

- When did the difficulty start? What was the child doing when it started? A sudden onset with fever and drooling suggests epiglottitis.
- Has the child ever had this problem before? What did the doctor say was wrong?
- What have you done for it? Does anything make it better or worse? Swollen air passages generally get better with cool air or mist. If medication has

been used, has it worked and how long has it been used?

- Is there a fever? A high fever usually occurs with epiglottitis, bacterial pneumonia, and bacterial meningitis.
- Is there a productive cough (e.g., does the child swallow frequently after coughing)? A productive cough indicates pneumonia.

### Assessment

- If wheezing is heard in only one lung area, suspect an inhaled foreign body.
- *Stridor with retractions is respiratory compromise.*
- Expiratory grunting (or whining) and nasal flaring indicate respiratory distress.
- An accurate assessment of respiratory effort in the infant or child can only be done with the shirt off.

***Difficulty Breathing in Absence of Stridor.**** Respiratory distress, shortness of breath, and asthma are common examples of difficulty breathing in absence of stridor. *Be prepared to deal with respiratory and cardiac arrest (see page 65)!* Monitor the respiratory status continuously. In children, be alert for signs of increasing respiratory distress. These may include decreased respiratory rate and/or depth, decreased breath sounds, cyanosis (late

*Modified from Manual for Emergency Medical Technicians. Emergency Medical Services Program. Albany: New York State Department of Health, 1990.

sign), visible soft tissue retractions, and decreased level of consciousness. *Be prepared to ventilate a sleepy, asthmatic child who has a silent chest!*

NOTE: Maintain a calm approach, and allow a child to assume a comfortable position or to be held by the parent, preferably in an upright position.

***Treatment****

1. Ensure that the patient's airway is open. If obstructed, see page 64.
2. Administer high-concentration oxygen, preferably humidified. Avoid agitating the child. Allow parent to hold the face mask, if tolerated, about six to eight inches from the child's face. Assist the patient's ventilations as necessary.
3. Obtain and record the vital signs, and repeat en route, as often as necessary.
4. Transport, keeping the patient warm.
5. Record all patient care information, including the medical history and treatment provided, on a prehospital care report.

***Difficulty Breathing with Stridor.**** Croup, epiglottitis, and barking cough are examples of difficulty breathing with stridor. Low fever, barking cough, or sternal retractions indicate croup. High fever, muffled voice, inability to swallow, or drooling indicate epiglottitis.

*Modified from Manual for Emergency Medical Technicians. Emergency Medical Services Program. Albany: New York State Department of Health, 1990.

### Treatment*

*If the child is conscious:*

1. Administer high-concentration oxygen, preferably humidified. Avoid agitating the child. Allow parent to hold the face mask, if tolerated, about six to eight inches from the child's face.
2. Transport the child calmly in an upright position (or in the parent's lap), keeping the child warm. *Do not force the child to lie down!* **Caution:** *Do not attempt to visualize the child's oropharynx!* Do not insert anything into the mouth or perform stressful procedures that could cause sudden, complete airway obstruction in these children!
3. Obtain and record the initial vital signs, including capillary refill—if tolerated and without agitating the child—and repeat en route as often as necessary.
4. Record all patient care information, including the medical history and treatment provided, on a prehospital care report.

*If the child is unconscious or becomes unconscious and is not breathing:*

1. Open the child's airway with the head-tilt–chin-lift maneuver.
2. Ventilate the child at a rate appropriate for the child's age (for neonate, 40/minute; <2 years, 20/minute; >2 years, 15/minute), using mouth-to-mouth or mouth-to-nose, pocket mask, or bag-

*Modified from Manual for Emergency Medical Technicians. Emergency Medical Services Program. Albany: New York State Department of Health, 1990.

valve-mask. *Make sure that the chest rises with each ventilation.*

NOTE: Adequate ventilation may require disabling the pop-off valve if the bag-valve-mask unit is so equipped.

3. Supplement ventilations with high-concentration oxygen.
4. Transport, keeping the child warm.
5. Obtain and record the initial vital signs, including capillary refill, and repeat en route as often as the situation indicates.
6. Record all patient care information, including the medical history and treatment provided, on a prehospital care report.

## Obstructed Airway

Management of an unconscious infant or child with a complete airway obstruction is the same as for the adult with one exception: the finger sweep is done only when the object is visualized.

### *Treatment*

1. If you are unable to ventilate the infant, try to reopen the airway and attempt a second ventilation.
2. If you are still unable to ventilate, administer four back blows and four chest thrusts.
3. Attempt to ventilate the infant at the end of each sequence. If you are unable to clear the airway after several attempts, rapid transport is essential to obtain surgical intervention.
4. If the airway is cleared, check the pulse and respirations and proceed accordingly. If there is a

pulse with no respirations, provide positive-pressure ventilation at the recommended rate.
5. If the infant has no pulse, perform CPR.

## Respiratory Arrest

Respiratory arrest in children is usually caused by a foreign body, mucus, or sudden infant death syndrome (SIDS).

***History.*** This is a very stressful time for all concerned; however, it is important to ask the following questions:

- What happened? Where did you find the child? If the infant was sleeping in bed, suspect SIDS.
- What was the child doing at the time? Was the child eating or choking? If eating or playing with small objects, suspect a foreign body obstructing the airway.

### *Assessment*

1. Note the presence of cyanosis or mottling.
2. If the child was in bed, note whether the bedsheet is stained with blood or vomitus.
3. Unless clear signs of death are present (rigor mortis or line of lividity), perform CPR and transport.
4. Note any bruises on the child. Suspect child abuse if bruises appear in various stages of healing.

NOTE: A line of lividity (blood pooling, usually in the extremities, ears, or flank) may resemble bruising but isn't.

5. *Do not question the parents in a suspicious manner.* If the possibility of abuse exists, law enforcement must be notified. Follow your service program's procedure.

### Treatment*

1. Establish airway and ventilation using basic life support techniques according to AHA/ARC standards.
   a. Open the airway using the head-tilt–chin-lift in the absence of trauma or the jaw-thrust maneuver if spinal injury is possible.
   b. Remove any *visible* airway obstruction by hand, and clear any accumulated secretions or fluids by suctioning. *Always be prepared to perform airway suctioning with suitable equipment as part of the primary survey!*
2. Immediately determine if the child is breathing adequately. If the child is cyanotic, the respiratory rate is low for the child's age, or capillary refill is less than 2 seconds:
   a. Ventilate at a rate appropriate for the child's age, using mouth-to-mouth or mouth-to-nose, pocket mask, or bag-valve-mask. *Make certain that the chest rises with each ventilation!*
   b. Supplement ventilations with high-concentration oxygen.
   c. Insert a proper-sized oropharyngeal airway if

*Modified from Manual for Emergency Medical Technicians. Emergency Medical Services Program. Albany: New York State Department of Health, 1990.

the gag reflex is absent. If it is present, insert a nasopharyngeal airway.

3. Identify and correct any remaining life-threatening conditions noted during the primary survey.
4. Transport, keeping the child warm.
5. Obtain and record the initial vital signs, and repeat en route as often as needed.
6. Record all patient care information, including the patient's medical history and all treatment provided, on a prehospital care report.

## Seizures

The most common cause of seizures in an infant or child is a rapid rise in temperature. The most common cause of sudden fever is an ear infection.

### *History*

- Has this ever happened before? What did the doctor say was wrong?
- What was the child doing when this started? If trauma is involved, see page 72. Overdose of several drugs can cause seizures, as can the failure to take epileptic medication.
- Has the child had a fever? Have you given the child anything for the fever? What, how much, and how often?

### *Assessment*

1. Carefully look for any rash, mottling, or concentric purple blotches. A rash, depending on where it is located and what it looks like, may indicate a viral infection (measles, roseola, or chicken

pox) or a bacterial infection (scarlet fever or meningitis). Mottling or purple blotches indicate a more serious problem. Follow the Communicable Disease Protocol on page 26.

2. Observe for a postseizure return to consciousness. A persistent altered level of consciousness is *not* normal and requires immediate transport.
3. Status epilepticus is defined as either a persistent seizure lasting for 20 minutes or recurrent seizures with no return to consciousness.
4. Observe for signs of trauma, abuse, or dehydration.

### *Special Assessment Considerations**

1. Establish and maintain airway control using basic life support techniques according to ARC/AHA standards.
2. Use caution when opening the airway of a pediatric patient. Do not hyperextend the infant's neck!
3. Protect the child from hurting himself or herself during the seizure.

***Treatment.**** If child has experienced trauma and is having a generalized tonic-clonic seizure, use cervical spine precautions. If trauma is not involved:

1. Place the child in the coma position unless airway or ventilatory maneuvers take priority.
2. Open the airway using the head-tilt–chin-lift or jaw-thrust maneuver, if possible. **Caution:** Do not force oral airways or other devices into the

*Modified from New York State Basic Life Support Protocols and New York City EMS Academy training protocols.

child's mouth if the teeth are tightly clenched. Use a nasopharyngeal airway instead, if needed.

3. Suction the airway as needed. Avoid stimulation of the posterior pharynx during suctioning, as this may cause vomiting.

NOTE: Be prepared to perform airway suctioning with suitable equipment as part of the expanded primary survey.

4. Administer high-concentration oxygen (preferably humidified) by a face mask. **Caution:** If ventilatory status is inadequate (the child is cyanotic, the respiratory rate is low for the child's age, or capillary refill is >2 seconds), initiate the respiratory distress or arrest protocol.
5. Transport, keeping the child warm. If child is febrile, try to cool with tepid water or wet towels. Do *not* cause the patient to shiver.
6. Obtain and record the initial vital signs, and repeat en route as often as needed.

## Shock

Hypovolemic shock (from dehydration or hemorrhage) is the most common type of shock in childhood. The next most common type is sepsis.

***History.*** Four or five episodes of diarrhea or vomiting and not voiding at least twice in 8 to 10 hours indicates dehydration in the infant or young child.

### *Assessment*

1. *Hypotension is a late sign of shock in a child.* A child can lose 50 percent of their blood supply

before hypotension occurs. The best indicators of early shock are an altered level of consciousness (ignores surroundings, minimal reaction to pain, failure to recognize parents), increased heart rate, and altered skin color and temperature.

NOTE: Relatively little blood loss can cause an infant or toddler to go into shock.

2. Children who have not reached puberty do not have the same sweating response to shock that an adult has. Many do not sweat or sweat only a little.
3. Tenting, dry mucous membranes, lack of urination, and sunken fontanelles (the soft spots in an infant's head) indicate hypovolemia from dehydration.

## PROTOCOL
## Noncardiogenic Shock in Children*

A cardiac cause for shock in children is rare. For the purpose of this protocol, pediatric shock is defined as signs of inadequate perfusion such as altered mental state (restlessness, inattention, confusion, agitation); tachycardia; weak or absent distal pulses; capillary refill >2 seconds; pallor; and cold, clammy, or mottled skin.

*Modified from Manual for Emergency Medical Technicians. Emergency Medical Services Program. Albany: New York State Department of Health, 1990.

- This protocol should be used even if the systolic blood pressure is normal or is difficult to obtain.
- A low systolic blood pressure means that the shock is severe.

### Treatment

1 Ensure that the patient's airway is open and that breathing and circulation are adequate.

NOTE: Manually stabilize the head and cervical spine if head or neck trauma is suspected!

2 Administer high-concentration oxygen, and be prepared to ventilate the patient!
3 Place the patient in a face-up position, and elevate the patient's legs 30 degrees.
4 If available, apply and inflate appropriate size MAST according to criteria for inflation (see page 73). Inflate the leg compartment until the pop-off valves pop open. Long leg air splints will accomplish the same purpose.

NOTE: If the abdominal section is inflated, the patient must be ventilated with a bag-valve-mask to assure adequate tidal volume.

- *Do not delay patient transport to apply and inflate MAST!*
- If the patient has an evisceration or an impaled object in the abdomen or legs, inflate

*Continued.*

only the MAST compartments *not* overlying the wound.
5 Obtain and record the vital signs, and repeat en route as often as the situation indicates (usually every 10 to 15 minutes).
6 Transport, keeping the patient warm. ■

## Trauma (Including Cardiac Arrest)
### *Assessment*

1. Bruises in various stages of healing are a sign of child abuse. Law enforcement must be notified. Follow your department's procedure.
2. Rib fractures are rare, but injury to the lung tissue from blunt trauma is not.
3. Children with head trauma have a high rate of organ system damage.
4. When assisting ventilations, *do not overventilate*. This can rupture the lungs and predispose the child to tension pneumothorax. *Make sure the chest rises with each ventilation.*

### *Treatment**

1. Establish and maintain airway control while manually stabilizing the cervical spine.
2. Assess the child's ventilatory status, including exposing the chest to locate and identify injuries.
   a. *If the ventilatory status is inadequate* (i.e.,

*Modified from Manual for Emergency Medical Technicians. Emergency Medical Services Program. Albany: New York State Department of Health, 1990.

cyanosis, respiratory rate low for child's age, or capillary refill >2 seconds):

(1) Ventilate the child at a rate appropriate for the child's age using mouth-to-mouth or mouth-to-nose, pocket mask, or bag-valve-mask.

(2) Seal any open chest wounds with Vaseline gauze, plastic, or other occlusive dressing.

(3) Supplement ventilations with high-concentration oxygen. **Caution:** Adequate ventilation may require disabling the pop-off valve if the bag-valve-mask unit is so equipped.

b. *If the ventilatory status is adequate,* administer high-concentration oxygen (preferably humidified) by a face mask as soon as possible.

3. Assess the child's circulatory status by palpating the brachial pulse in infants and the carotid pulse in children.

a. If *pulse is absent* (traumatic cardiac arrest):

(1) Initiate transport immediately while performing CPR.

(2) Take appropriate steps to control hemorrhage.

(3) Either inflate the leg compartments of an appropriately sized MAST or elevate the foot of the backboard 30 degrees if MAST are not available.

b. If *pulse is present:*

(1) Search for any life-threatening hemorrhage and test capillary refill.

(2) Initiate transport immediately while as-

sessing the circulatory status. *If shock is present* (i.e., tachycardia, capillary refill >2 seconds, cold clammy skin, thirst, restlessness, and/or hypotension), either inflate appropriately sized MAST or elevate the foot of the backboard 30 degrees if MAST are not available.

(3) Keep the child warm en route.

(4) Obtain and record the initial vital signs, including capillary refill, and repeat en route as often as needed.

c. *If life-threatening hemorrhage is present:*

(1) Initiate transport immediately while taking appropriate steps to control hemorrhage.

NOTE: Relatively small amounts of blood loss may be life-threatening in small children.

(2) If shock is present, see b. (2) above.

(3) If head injury is suspected, the child is not alert, the arms and legs are abnormally flexed and/or extended (neurologic posturing), the child is seizing, or has a GCS score <8 (see page 224), hyperventilate the child with high-concentration oxygen (usually at a rate of 30/minute).

d. As for all runs, record all patient care information, including the medical history and treatment provided, on a prehospital care report.

## PREGNANCY AND RELATED PROBLEMS

Women undergo extensive physiologic changes during pregnancy, especially after the first trimester. A pregnant woman can lose one-third of her total blood supply before changes in vital signs are noticed.

Survival of the baby depends on survival of the mother. Aggressive treatment for the mother is aggressive treatment for the baby.

### *Treatment Priorities*

1. Oxygenation, spinal precautions, and controlling hemorrhage take priority.
2. Airway management must be aggressive. Oxygen consumption is greatly increased because of fetal demands and upward displacement of the diaphragm.
3. Assume the stomach is full, and prepare for vomiting.
4. Control hemorrhage with direct pressure. Apply sanitary pads for vaginal bleeding.
5. Administer high-concentration oxygen by mask nonrebreather. If ventilations are inadequate or inefficient, assist with bag-valve-mask.
6. If shock is present, refer immediately to Shock Protocol, page 153.

NOTE: Signs of shock may not be readily apparent, the mechanism of injury is the most important indicator. If mechanism meets trauma center criteria, the mother should always be transported whether or not obvious signs of injury are present. **CAUTION:** *Use only legs of MAST.*

7. Pregnant patients should always be transported on their *left* side or sitting up. Elevate the left side of the backboard.
8. Keep patient warm during transport. Repeat and record vital signs en route as often as necessary (at least every 15 minutes). Record all patient care information and treatment provided on a prehospital care report.

### *Special Considerations*

- Mark the top of the fundus (uterus) with a pen and reassess every 10 to 15 minutes. Expansion of the fundus indicates internal bleeding.
- An abdominal bruise, especially in the presence of pain, may indicate uterine rupture or placental separation.
- Be prepared for premature rupture of membranes and labor. If delivery is imminent, turn on the heat in the ambulance to provide warm environment for the baby.

## Childbirth

Deciding whether to transport or to stay and deliver the baby can be determined by answers to the following questions:

- Is this your first pregnancy?
  —First pregnancies usually take longer—up to an hour of hard labor before actual delivery. Subsequent deliveries are shorter and unpredictable. Ask if previous deliveries were long or short. If the patient has had a C-section in the past, transport immediately to the hospital.
  —Don't be embarrassed to have the mother re-

move her underwear with the onset of what she thinks is labor.

- What time did your contractions begin, and how far apart are they?
  - —Pains get closer together as labor progresses until they are 2 to 3 minutes apart and regular.

NOTE: To determine how far apart the contractions are, time from the end of one to the beginning of the next. The *duration* of a contraction is timed from the beginning to the end of the same contraction.

- Has your water broken?
  - —Rupture along with contractions indicates actual labor is taking place; however, *delivery may not necessarily be imminent.*
- Do you have the urge to move your bowels?
  - —If yes, check for a presenting part. If it is the head, prepare for delivery. If it is the umbilical cord or a limb, see Special Considerations, page 78, item 4.
- Have you had bleeding or a bloody show?
  - —If yes, small amounts (about 250 mL) is normal. Active bleeding or large clots may indicate a serious problem, such as placenta previa. Transport immediately.
- When is your due date?
  - —If the mother is more than 2 weeks early, contact the hospital so the nursery can prepare for a possible premature baby.
  - —If the baby is premature, delivery may be rapid. See Special Care for the Premature Baby, page 81.
- Have you had any problems with this pregnancy?

Do you have any medical problems? Do you take any medications?
—Diabetic mothers should be transported immediately.
—Mothers with pregnancy-induced hypertension or preeclampsia need special care and calm transport (no lights or sirens).
—If the patient is in **early labor** (irregular and mild pains with no urge to push, membranes not ruptured, and no bloody show), it is not necessary to check for a presenting part.

### *Special Considerations*

1. If the mother's water has broken, ask what it looked like. Meconium staining (greenish) indicates there may be a problem with the baby. Be prepared to suction infant repeatedly and to resuscitate.
2. If the patient is in **late labor** (regular contractions 1 to 2 minutes apart with an urge to push, ruptured membranes, and bloody show), check for a presenting part. If crowning is present (i.e., a presenting part is visible), prepare for delivery.
3. If an arm, leg, or buttocks are the presenting part, turn the mother on her left side, elevate the hips, administer high-concentration oxygen, and transport to the hospital immediately.
4. If the umbilical cord is the presenting part, *DO NOT allow her to sit.* Assist her to a knee-chest position or elevate the hips with pillows. Apply high-concentration oxygen, then with your gloved hand follow the cord up to the presenting part and elevate the presenting part off the cord. Maintain this position en route to the hospital.

5. After delivery, the most important thing you can do is to clear the airway and keep the baby warm by giving the baby to the mother.
6. The newborn must also be assessed. The most common method is by using the Apgar Scoring Chart (Table 3–1 on page 90).

### Normal Birthing Procedure

1. Wash hands if there is time, then position and drape the mother, and prepare a sterile field. *Do not leave the mother unattended to perform any of these tasks*. The second EMT should lay out clean towels and infant resuscitation equipment in a warm area nearby.
2. Apply gentle counterpressure to the crown of the baby's head to prevent an explosive delivery. Ask the mother to pant like a dog so that pushing is controlled.
3. Once the head is delivered, tell the mother not to push while you check for the cord around the baby's neck. If a tight cord is found (one that cannot be easily slipped around the baby's head), place two clamps very close together on the cord and cut the cord now.
4. If there is meconium-stained fluid, quickly wipe the baby's face with gauze to remove excess meconium; then suction the baby's mouth and nose with a bulb syringe before proceeding with the delivery. The mouth is always suctioned first because suction of the nose could elicit a gasp and the baby would aspirate the meconium inside the mouth.
5. Ask the mother to push as you give gentle trac-

tion if necessary to deliver the shoulders (downward traction for the anterior shoulder and upward traction for the posterior shoulder).

6. Suction with a bulb syringe when the infant is delivered.
7. Clamp and cut the cord if it has not already been cut. Examine the stump of the cord to make sure there is no bleeding.
8. Place the infant on towels for resuscitation.
9. When the placenta has separated, the uterus will form in a hard ball and there will be lengthening of the cord. Ask the mother to bear down while the placenta is delivered. Do not pull on the cord.
10. Place a warm blanket on the mother and observe the fundus of her uterus while transporting her to the hospital. Massage the uterus when necessary to prevent hemorrhage.

### Resuscitation of the Newborn

1. Dry the infant and place on a clean towel in a warm place. *Keep the infant warm.* Temperature should be between 80° F to 90° F, or hot enough to make you sweat.
2. Position the infant with the neck only slightly extended (so the airway is not blocked by hyperextension).
3. Suction the mouth and then the nose with a bulb syringe.
4. Stimulate by rubbing the infant's back or slapping the feet.
5. Evaluate breathing.
6. Repeat step 4 twice only if the infant is apneic at this point.

7. If the infant is still not breathing, give positive-pressure ventilation with bag-valve-mask and 100 percent oxygen.
8. Evaluate the heart rate after 15 to 30 seconds of positive-pressure ventilation.
9. If the heart rate is less than 60 or between 60 and 80 but not increasing, begin chest compressions ½ to ¾ of an inch at 120 compressions per minute.
10. After 30 seconds of chest compressions, check the heart rate for 6 seconds. If below 80, continue both chest compressions and positive-pressure ventilation. If heart rate is >80, proceed to step 11.
11. Evaluate color. If the infant is now pink, continue to observe. If cyanotic, administer 100 percent oxygen. Continue to evaluate breathing, heart rate, and color during transportation to the hospital.

### Special Care for the Premature Baby

1. Dry and wrap the baby snugly in a warm blanket; keep the head covered to reduce heat loss. As added protection, an outer layer of plastic wrap or aluminum foil can be used. Be sure to keep the outer wrap away from the baby's face.
2. Follow the procedure for resuscitation of newborn, if necessary.
3. The mother should be allowed to hold her infant. This aids in keeping the infant warm and promotes the bonding process.
4. Provide 100 percent oxygen and positive-pressure ventilation as needed. These babies have

immature lungs and are prone to respiratory distress.

5. Do not allow premature babies of less than 34 weeks' gestation to nurse. They cannot coordinate sucking, breathing, and swallowing and are prone to aspiration.
6. Handle very gently. Premature babies are prone to intracranial hemorrhage and other injuries. The blood volume of a very premature infant is only a few ounces, so even a slight loss can lead to shock.
7. Avoid exposing the premature infant to any potential source of infection.
8. The baby should be transported in a prewarmed ambulance with a temperature of between 90° F and 100° F. Turn off the air-conditioning in the warmer months.
9. Radio ahead and advise the hospital that you are transporting a premature baby.
10. Provide rapid transport.

## Preeclampsia / Eclampsia

Common chief complaints include: headache, difficulty breathing, swelling, abdominal pain, and blurred vision. The onset of seizures in a preeclamptic mother classifies her as eclamptic. In the absence of labor, the following are key questions:

- Have you had any problems with this pregnancy?
- Do you have any medical problems? Diabetic mothers are prone to preeclampsia / eclampsia and should be transported immediately. Epileptic mothers may have seizures caused by their epilepsy. Unless the EMT can identify the mother as an epileptic (e.g., by a Medic Alert necklace), he

or she may mistakenly think that the mother is eclamptic.

- Do you take any medications? Mothers taking diuretics ("water pills") or antihypertensives ("blood pressure pills") are most likely to suffer from preeclampsia/eclampsia.

The following questions may be necessary depending on the situation:

- Have you had any prenatal care? Mothers without any prenatal care are more likely to have problems, including preeclampsia/eclampsia.
- Do you take drugs recreationally? Mothers who take street drugs are more likely to have premature births and problem pregnancies with difficult deliveries.

### *Assessment*

1. Suspect preeclampsia/eclampsia if the patient has hypertension (diastolic >90) and a puffy look.
2. Pulmonary edema may be present.
3. Photophobia (sensitivity to light) and/or fine muscle tremors are warning signs that a seizure may be imminent.
4. Preventing stimulation (e.g., not using flashing lights and sirens) helps to control seizures.

### *Treatment*

1. Control the airway; administer high-concentration oxygen; have suction ready.
2. Transport in an upright position if patient has difficulty breathing; otherwise, position on left side.

3. Provide quiet, dark environment; avoid unnecessary jostling or noise.

NOTE: Keep patient calm; *don't use lights or sirens during transport.*

4. If a seizure occurs, follow protocol on page 130.

## Vaginal/Perineal Bleeding

Treatment of severe vaginal bleeding, regardless of the cause, focuses on the prevention of shock. It is important to find out if vaginal bleeding is from miscarriage, postpartum hemorrhage, perineal trauma, or postdelivery wound separation.

### *Treatment*

1. Control the patient's airway; apply high-concentration oxygen.
2. Place in a supine position with legs elevated. If the patient is 6 or more months pregnant, place on left side.
3. If possible, attempt to control the bleeding.
   - *Miscarriage.* Collect any expelled tissue and bring it to hospital with patient. Place sanitary pad over perineal area.
   - *Postpartum hemorrhage.* Massage the uterus, and put the baby to breast.
   - *Perineal trauma.* Apply direct pressure with a soft sterile dressing or sanitary pad. An ice pack applied to the site may slow bleeding and provide some pain relief.
   - *Postdelivery wound separation.* Apply direct pressure with a soft sterile dressing or sanitary pad. Bleeding is considered excessive if more than five pads become saturated.

4. If shock is present follow Shock Protocol, page 153. If MAST are used, inflate only the legs.

## PATIENTS WITH TUBES AND SHUNTS

EMTs often encounter patients with tubes and shunts who require special care when transporting. Six common types are described here:

1. **Urinary catheters.** These are common in persons who have lost bladder control (nursing home residents, paraplegics, and quadriplegics). Have attendants drain the bag before transport, if possible. If not, keep the bag lower than the level of the bladder to prevent urine from flowing back into the patient.
2. **Central line catheters.** These catheters are found in the upper chest and are inserted into a major vessel that drains directly into the heart or superior vena cava. They are used for administering medications or in hyperalimentation. These catheters must be clamped closed and secured before transport to prevent any tension on them. If bleeding occurs at the site, apply direct pressure.
3. **Feeding tubes.** Feeding tubes are usually through the nose and should be clamped closed and secured to prevent any tension on them.
4. **Hydrocephalic shunt.** These tubes are placed in a brain ventricle and threaded down behind the ear through the neck and into the abdomen to drain the excess fluid caused by hydrocephalus. A small bubble can be palpated just under the scalp. The shunt may plug, which may result

in signs and symptoms of increased intracranial pressure (e.g., vomiting and seizures). If this occurs, transport the patient to a hospital familiar with such devices (usually a children's hospital). Protect the site from trauma.

5. **Kidney dialysis shunt.** These shunts are found in the lower arm, usually close to the wrist. Protect the site from any trauma. Never take a blood pressure in the arm with a shunt. If bleeding occurs at the site, apply direct pressure.
   - Abdominal, or peritoneal, dialysis is also common. The connection site is in the abdomen and usually is connected to a fluid-containing bag. Do *not* dislodge bags. Protect the site from pulling and other trauma.
6. **Tracheostomy tubes.** These are usually permanent openings into the trachea. Occasionally, a tracheostomy will have a trach-tube in place. Do not dislodge or remove unless obstructed. Obstruction is usually due to a mucous plug. Manually removing the plug by suctioning with a sterile, flexible catheter is usually all that is necessary.

## STREET PEOPLE

In urban areas, squad calls frequently involve street people or alcoholics. Reasons for the calls vary from seeking a warm hospital bed to being the victim of a brutal assault or suffering from a chronic subdural bleed.

### *Special Considerations*

- Street people may be abusive and combative, posing a physical threat to the EMT.
- There is a tendency to ignore or discount complaints or to take shortcuts because of their body odor, unconventional behavior, or frequency of encounters. Always perform a complete assessment, especially a thorough neurologic assessment. EMTs are more likely to err or use poor judgment with street people.
- Remember to take precautions for airborne and bloodborne diseases.
- Alcoholics get sick too. Remember these precautions:
  - —Pain sensations may be suppressed or distorted; localizing the area of pain may be difficult.
  - —An assessment may reveal old untreated injuries; open wounds are often infected.
  - —A minor blow to the head may be life-threatening because of the tendency for subdural bleeds.
  - —Alcoholics also may have a head injury or be hypoglycemic, both of which mimic intoxication.
  - —Gastrointestinal bleeds and varicose veins in the esophagus are common. Do not use an esophageal obturator airway on alcoholics. Use an oral airway with bag-valve-mask instead.

## ELDERLY PATIENTS

The elderly often have coexisting medical problems that may have caused the trauma or complicate the injury (e.g., a heart attack that causes a fall). In an elderly diabetic, hypoglycemia may mimic a head injury, or vice versa. *History-taking is extremely important in the elderly*. Among other things, the use of antihypertensive drugs such as propranolol (Inderal) and timolol maleate (Blocadren), may mask tachycardias and prevent sweating, vasoconstriction, and so on. Bring all medications to the hospital with the patient.

### Treatment Priorities

1. Maintain an airway, especially if the patient is vomiting.
2. Administer high-concentration oxygen if there are signs of altered mental status or shock. *Oxygen should never be withheld* from patients requiring it, even if they have COPD.
3. If shock is present, see page 153.
4. Keep patient warm during transport. Repeat and record vital signs en route as often as necessary. Record all patient care information and treatment provided on a prehospital care report.

### Special Considerations

- Arthritic changes may make certain positions difficult or painful. Ensure a comfortable position, whenever possible.
- If curvature of the spine is obvious, transport patient on side. If a backboard is necessary, pad the open areas for support and comfort, and elevate the left side of the board. If metal backboards are used, blanket them first for warmth.
- Do not assume a joint deformity is arthritis. Compare the joint on the other side, and if in doubt,

treat as a fracture or dislocation. Loss of range-of-motion may be a result of arthritis.

- Always assume that hip pain is a fracture until proven otherwise. The classic external rotation and shortening is not always present in the elderly.
- Falls on flexed knees also may cause femur fractures. Falls on outstretched arms may cause elbow fractures or shoulder injuries.
- The skin of older persons may be very fragile. When bandaging, tape dressing to dressing, *not* dressing to skin.
- A blood pressure of 110/70 may be *hypo*tensive in a normally *hyper*tensive older person. Treat your patient holistically, and do not depend on any one vital sign.
- The elderly are extremely sensitive to hypoxia, hypotension, hypoglycemia, and hypothermia.
- Be sensitive to concerns of the patient or spouse (e.g., lock up the house when you leave), make certain that glasses and dentures are taken, and enlist neighbors to look after pets.

**TABLE 3–1 ■ Apgar Score**

| Characteristic Evaluated | Score | | |
|---|---|---|---|
| | 0 | 1 | 2 |
| Appearance (color) | Blue or pale | Body pink, extremities blue | Completely pink |
| Pulse rate | Absent | $<100$ | $>100$ |
| Grimace (reflex irritability) | No response | Grimace | Cough or sneeze |
| Activity (muscle tone) | Limp | Some flexion of extremities | Active movement |
| Respiratory effort | Absent | Slow or irregular | Good cry |

From Apgar V.A., A proposal for a new method of evaluation of the newborn infant, *Current Research in Anesthesia and Analgesia* 32:260–267, 1953.

# CHIEF COMPLAINT OR INJURY

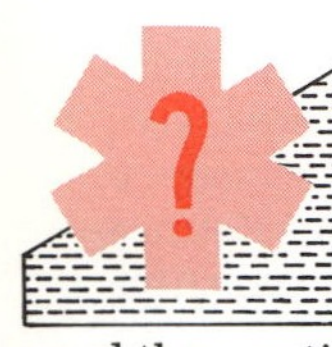

## ABDOMINAL EMERGENCIES

The most dangerous abdominal emergency is one that requires rapid surgical intervention. The following points are geared toward these patients.

**Nausea** and **vomiting** are common but nonspecific symptoms. Check what position the patient is in. If supine or lying on side with knees raised and shallow breathing or guarding, suspect an **acute abdomen,** particularly with distention and tenderness. However, if the patient is a woman of childbearing age, assess for shock and suspect a ruptured **ovarian cyst** or **tubal pregnancy.** Specific questions include:

- Have you been vomiting? What does it look like (e.g., coffee grounds, bright or dark blood, or partially digested food)?

- Do you have diarrhea? What do your stools look like? Black and tarry stools indicate digested blood; if they resemble red currant jelly, suspect bleeding in the colon. Blood in the gastrointestinal (GI) tract has a distinctive foul odor.
- Do you have other problems along with the abdominal pain? Fainting or syncope may indicate serious internal bleeding.
- Does the pain stay in one place or radiate to other areas:
  —Free blood in the peritoneal cavity radiates to either shoulder or neck.
  —**Gall bladder** problems radiate pain to the right scapula, right shoulder, or across the epigastrium.
  —**Kidney stones** radiate pain to the groin.
  —Abdominal **aneurysms** radiate pain to the back, either side, or one or both legs. Look for a pulsating mass, although not all patients with an aneurysm have this.
  —Blood in the capsule of the spleen radiates pain to the left shoulder or neck.
  —Blood in the liver capsule radiates pain to the right shoulder or neck.

### Treatment of Abdominal Emergencies (Without Trauma)

1. *Maintain an airway,* especially in the presence of vomiting. Patients with altered mental status and vomiting should be placed in the left lateral recumbent position, with suction on standby to aid in keeping the airway clear en route.
2. *Administer high-concentration oxygen* if there

are signs of shock or peritonitis (to compensate for the associated shallow breathing).

3. *Treat shock if present.* Maintain body temperature, elevate legs, and consider using the MAST.
4. *Place the patient in a position of comfort* if this is not contraindicated by the need to control the airway or treat the patient for shock. Patients with peritoneal signs may find the most comfort by being transported supine, or on their side, with hips and knees flexed. A pillow may be placed under the knees to support the weight of the legs.
5. *Give nothing by mouth.* The patient with an abdominal emergency may require surgery, and a full stomach adds to the risk of aspiration when anesthesia is administered.
6. *Complete your examination while en route to the hospital.* Repeat vital signs as indicated. Record your findings. Notify the hospital of your impending arrival with a critical patient.

## ALLERGY/ANAPHYLAXIS

Anaphylaxis is a severe allergic reaction. Signs and symptoms vary greatly, but shock, bronchoconstriction, and airway obstruction are common. Onset can be extremely rapid or up to an hour or more later.

A detailed history—specifically asking about past exposures to insect stings, for example—is very important. In the absence of a known allergen, assessment findings are the only clue. Look for an Epi-Pen (self-injectable epinephrine).

General flushing, hives, itching, or blotching, especially with shortness of breath or difficult breathing, is common. **Hives** are not always present. Internal or subcutaneous hives result in pain and swelling (without blotching) of the extremities.

Eyes and mucous membranes may swell before any redness or hives form. An ingested allergen, such as shellfish, may cause extreme vomiting and diarrhea simultaneously.

### *Treatment**

1. Ensure that the patient's airway is open and that breathing and circulation are adequate, and suction as necessary.
2. Assist the patient in self-administration of prescribed epinephrine if he or she has an anaphylaxis (bee-sting) kit.
3. Transport the patient immediately in a position of comfort, while keeping the patient warm, providing reassurance, and loosening tight clothing.
4. Administer high-concentration oxygen and assist ventilations if necessary.
5. If ventilatory status is inadequate, refer to pages 50–52.
6. Assess for shock. If shock is present, refer immediately to page 153.
7. If cardiac arrest occurs, perform CPR according to AHA/ARC Standards.
8. Obtain and record the initial vital signs, and repeat en route as often as the situation indi-

*Modified from Manual for Emergency Medical Technicians. Emergency Medical Services Program. Albany: New York State Department of Health, 1990.

cates. *Be alert for changes in the level of consciousness!*

9. If the patient is a child, maintain a calm approach to both the child and parent. Allow the child to assume and maintain a position of comfort or to be held by the parent, preferably in an upright position.

## ALTERED MENTAL STATUS

A patient with altered mental status without trauma and respiratory or cardiovascular complications may present in many ways (e.g., with anxiety, confusion, or combativeness). Because altered mental status may be attributed to many different causes, it is important to perform a thorough assessment and to check for Medic Alert necklace, bracelet, anklet, or wallet card. Usually clues at the scene, a history, and initial assessment findings will indicate which protocol to follow. Try to answer the following questions:

- What happened?
  - —A sudden collapse while eating may indicate an **obstructed airway;** a sudden collapse at other times may indicate cardiac problems or stroke.
  - —Sudden confusion, inability to talk, altered gait, or odd behavior may be **stroke** symptoms.
  - —Exposure to fertilizers, insecticides, or toxic chemicals may cause **poisoning.** Look for containers.
  - —If the patient was at a party, suspect ethanol intoxication or **drug overdose** (check for track marks).

- Does the patient have any medical problems? What medications are they taking?
  - —A history of heart problems or high blood pressure may indicate a cardiac problem or stroke.
  - —A history of **diabetes** may indicate a diabetic reaction.
  - —A history of **seizures** may indicate that the person is in a postseizure state. Common home medications for epileptics include phenobarbital (Solfoton), carbamazepine (Tegretol), primidone (Mysoline), and valproic acid (Depakene). A common side effect is hypertrophied gums. Bruises or abrasions on the tongue also implicate seizure, but not all seizures result in incontinence.
  - —A history of **allergies,** especially to insect bites and stings if the patient is outdoors, warrants checking the body for welts. Check the pockets for an Epi-Pen (self-injectable epinephrine). General flushing, hives, or blotched skin, especially in the presence of shortness of breath or difficult breathing, indicates an allergic reaction.
- Any complaints of pain or discomfort before this incident?
  - —A **headache** may indicate increasing intracranial pressure. Check pupils for reaction and equality. Check blood pressure for hypertension.
  - —Indigestion or abdominal pain before unconsciousness in persons over age 30 may indicate a **cardiac problem** or **GI bleeding.** Ask about vomiting and what it looked like. Ask about stools or check undergarments for traces of

black, tarry stool. Check for signs and symptoms of shock, and if present, follow Shock Protocol on page 153. If cardiogenic shock is suspected, note page 155. It is important to differentiate between shock caused by internal bleeding and cardiogenic shock by listening to the lung sounds. A patient with internal bleeding has clear lung sounds, but a patient in cardiogenic shock may have diminished lung sounds, wheezes, or crackles (rales). If an irregular pulse is present, suspect a cardiac problem.

### *Treatment**

NOTE: These instructions are for patients who are verbally responsive, respond to painful stimuli, or are unresponsive.

1. Ensure that the patient's airway is open and that breathing and circulation are adequate, and suction as necessary.
2. Administer high-concentration oxygen. In children, humidified oxygen is preferred.
3. Obtain and record the vital signs, including determining the patient's level of consciousness.
4. If the patient is **unresponsive or responds only to painful stimuli**, transport immediately, keeping the patient warm.
5. If the patient is **diabetic and is conscious, has**

*From Manual for Emergency Medical Technicians. Emergency Medical Services Program. Albany: New York State Department of Health, 1990.

**a gag reflex, and is able to drink without assistance**, provide glucose or a sugar solution (if available) by mouth, then transport, keeping the patient warm.

6. Repeat and record the vital signs, including the level of consciousness and GCS score en route as often as necessary (see pages 42–43).

## BEHAVIORAL EMERGENCIES

Behavioral problems may be acute or chronic, temporary or permanent. Problems may occur with communication, situations, or personal prejudices. The following suggestions may be helpful.

- *Your safety comes first,* call law enforcement if you suspect any potential or actual threat exists.
- If restraints are used, assess and record motor and sensory reflexes and circulation to the restrained extremity(ies) every 15 minutes.
- Some medical problems mimic behavioral emergencies. Look for such clues as insulin, syringes, prescription bottles, Medic Alert tags, Vial-of-Life in the refrigerator, food-drug reactions, signs of trauma, or pills laying around (drug overdose). Complete a history and physical assessment as much as possible.
- People with chronic psychiatric problems get sick too. A paranoid schizophrenic, for example, may describe his chest pain in delusional terms: "They are shooting darts into my chest."
- Maintain a calm approach. Many anxiety reactions can be effectively managed by talking the person down.

***Assessment.*** Assessment of patients with behavioral emergencies includes both a physical and emotional assessment. The emotional assessment is done after the physical and consists of the following steps. For attempted suicide, see page 134.

NOTE: A physical assessment may not always be possible to do.

1. **Behavior.** What is the patient doing now? What was the patient doing that resulted in the call? Are activities threatening to the patient or others (e.g., walking in the middle of traffic).
2. **Emotion.** Is the emotion appropriate? Does the person refuse to look at you? Does the emotion match what they say (e.g., laughing while telling you how depressed they feel).
3. **Thinking.** Can they tell you what happened today with a logical order or progression, or do they go off on tangents? Are they oriented to place and time? Remember that street people do not always know what day it is and may not know or care, who the president is. (See page 34.)
4. **Hallucinations.** Are the patient's thoughts based in reality? If the patient is hallucinating, find out whether he or she is hearing voices, for example, or seeing things. If the patient is hearing voices, ask what the voices are saying. The answer is one of the best indications of a potential threat to you or others.

***Treatment.*** Treatment is supportive.

## CHEST (Cardiac) PAIN

Any patient who complains of chest pain or discomfort, especially in those over age 40, should be suspected of having a cardiac problem until proven otherwise. Remember that even people in their 20s have heart attacks. Page 102 gives the protocol for respiratory or cardiac arrest. See also Defibrillation, page 103.

- Breaking out in a **cold sweat, shortness of breath, dizziness,** and **nausea** and vomiting are all indicators of a cardiac problem, especially in the presence of chest pain or discomfort.
- Pain may radiate to a shoulder, either side of the neck, and down the left arm or hand.
- Pain is not always present. If present, the patient may describe a crushing or **squeezing sensation** or complain of **indigestion.**
- **Diabetics** have a high incidence of "silent" heart attacks. Signs and symptoms include breaking out in a cold sweat, dizziness, and a worsening of symptoms on exertion in the absence of chest pain.
- An **irregular pulse** in the presence of syncope or dizziness indicates a cardiac problem.
- A comfortable position for the patient may require elevating the head and chest to aid breathing.
- Several conditions mimic heart attack: gall bladder problems, inner ear syndrome, and hiatal hernia. However, *in the adult, always suspect heart attack* if any signs and symptoms are present.

### *Treatment**

1. Ensure that the patient's airway is open and that breathing and circulation are adequate. **Caution:** Be prepared to deal with respiratory and cardiac arrest (see page 102).
2. Administer high-concentration oxygen. Be prepared to assist ventilations with bag-valve-mask.
3. Place the patient in a comfortable position while providing reassurance and loosening tight clothing.
4. Obtain and record the vital signs, and repeat en route as often as necessary (at least every 15 minutes).
5. Transport, keeping the patient warm.
6. Record all patient care information, including the patient's medical history and all treatment provided, on a prehospital care report.
7. If chest pain is present and if the patient has a prescription for sublingual nitroglycerin and a systolic blood pressure of ≥90 mm Hg, the EMT may help the patient self-administer the medicine as indicated on the container.

*Modified from Manual for Emergency Medical Technicians. Emergency Medical Services Program. Albany: New York State Department of Health, 1990.

## PROTOCOL
## Respiratory or Cardiac Arrest

1 Provide BLS according to AHA/ARC standards
   - *If ventilations are unsuccessful, refer immediately to the obstructed airway protocol.*

2 Insert an oropharyngeal or nasopharyngeal airway if the gag reflex is absent.

3 Ventilate with an adjunctive device and high-concentration oxygen.

***Minimum Rate of Ventilation***

| | |
|---|---|
| Adults | 12/min |
| Children ≥2 yrs | 15/min |
| Children <2 yrs | 20/min |

   - Assure that the chest rises with each ventilation!
   - If chest doses not rise, suspect destruction. If airway is clear, suspect increased pressure in the lungs (i.e., bronchospasm, fluid, tension pneumothorax, etc.).

4 Evaluate the effectiveness of the ventilations/compressions.

5 Transport *immediately,* keeping the patient warm.

6 Record all patient care information, including the patient's medical history and all treatment provided, on a Prehospital Care Report. ■

From Manual of Emergency Medical Technicians. Emergency Medical Services Program. Albany: New York State Department of Health, 1990.

## DEFIBRILLATION

### Automatic/Semiautomatic Defibrillation

The following generic procedure can be used for most automatic and semiautomatic defibrillators. To decide when defibrillation is needed, see the following Protocol or follow your agency's policies.

### PROTOCOL
### Defibrillation of Patients with Cardiac Arrest and Ventricular Fibrillation or Ventricular Tachycardia

1 Begin CPR (if you witness cardiac arrest, give a precordial thump if a defibrillator is not immediately available).
2 As soon as a monitor–defibrillator is available, evaluate rhythm.
3 If ventricular fibrillation or ventricular tachycardia is observed, and no pulse, defibrillate at 200 J.
4 Reassess pulse and rhythm; if no pulse and if ventricular fibrillation or ventricular tachycardia is still present, defibrillate at 200 to 300 J.
5 Reassess pulse and rhythm; if no pulse and if ventricular fibrillation or ventricular tachy-

*Continued.*

cardia is still present, defibrillate at 360 or 400 J.

6 Reassess pulse and rhythm; continue CPR if necessary.

7 If cardiac arrest persists, perform CPR for 1 minute and perform up to three more defibrillations at 360 J.

8 Follow local strategy to obtain earliest ALS. ■

### *Procedure**

1. If no respirations and pulse are detected, begin CPR (Fig. 4–1).
2. Attach the electrodes and turn on the device.
3. Press the button to analyze the rhythm. No one should be in contact with the patient while the machine analyzes the rhythm.
4. If ventricular fibrillation is present, the machine automatically charges to 200 J while sounding an audible alarm or voice recording directing bystanders to stand clear.
5. The machine then advises you to press the defibrillation button.
6. Make sure that everyone is clear of the patient and deliver the shock. Say, "I'm clear, you're clear, everybody's clear," while carefully observing the area around the patient.
7. Following the shock, push the analyze button.

*Modified from Manual for Emergency Medical Technicians. Emergency Medical Services Program. Albany: New York State Department of Health, 1990.

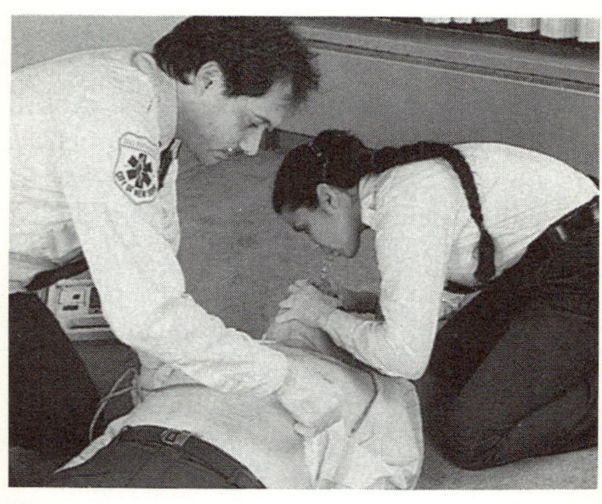

**Figure 4–1** Placement of Fast-Patch electrodes for a semiautomatic, automatic, or manual defibrillation.
*Illustration continued on following page*

8. If the machine advises another shock, repeat steps 5 through 7 above.
9. If ventricular fibrillation persists, the energy level can be set between 200 and 300 J for the next defibrillation and increased to 360 J for the third shock, if necessary.
10. The sequence of three shocks is repeated as necessary, usually with 1 minute of CPR in between the sequences.

## Manual Defibrillation

The following generic procedure can be used with most manual defibrillators. To decide when defi-

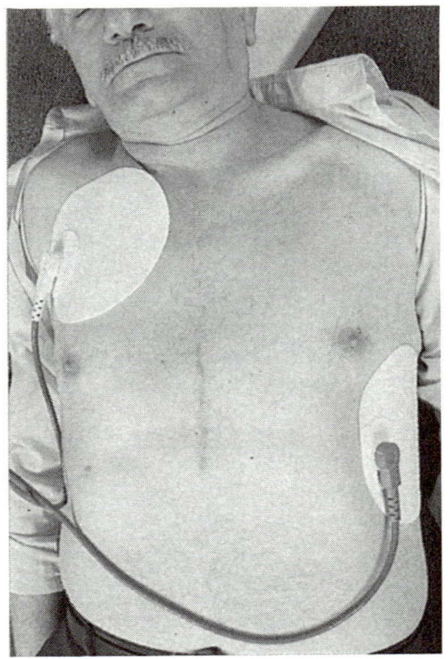

**Figure 4–1** *Continued*

brillation is needed, see pages 103–104 or follow your agency's policies.

### Procedure

1. If no respirations and pulse are detected, initiate CPR.
2. As soon as the monitor-defibrillator is available, attach leads and turn on the recorder and the medical control recording device.

3. Apply paddles to correct location, using conductive gel and firm (25-pound) pressure, or use Fast-Patch electrodes.
4. Operator announces, "Stand clear," and makes sure no one is in contact with the patient, stretcher, or equipment.
5. Press the discharge buttons on the paddles to defibrillate.
6. Reevaluate pulse and rhythm.
7. If the patient is still in ventricular fibrillation, repeat steps 3 to 7 with 200 to 300 J.
8. If the patient is still in ventricular fibrillation, repeat steps 3 to 7 with 360 J.
9. If the rhythm changes, always evaluate the need for CPR.

## COLD EXPOSURE

Children and the elderly are most susceptible to cold-related injuries. The two types of cold exposure are general (hypothermia) and local (frostbite).

### Hypothermia

***History.*** The levels of hypothermia are shown in Table 4–1. Exposure to cold air or water immersion is an important variable. Children often have a better outcome in cold water immersion than adults. Wind chill factors significantly increase the risk of exposure (Table 4–2).

Remember that hypothermia can occur at relatively mild temperatures. Hypovolemia, alcohol and drug intoxication, hypoglycemia, malnutrition, and

**TABLE 4–1 ■ Levels of Hypothermia**

| Temperature (° C) | (° F) | Signs and Symptoms |
|---|---|---|
| **MILD** | | |
| 35 | 95 | Shivering begins |
| 34 | 93.2 | Amnesia |
| 33 | 91.4 | Poor muscular coordination |
| **MODERATE** | | |
| 32 | 89.6 | Stupor |
| 31 | 87.8 | Shivering stops |
| 30 | 86 | Irregular heart rhythms |
| 29 | 85.2 | Further loss of consciousness<br>Pupils dilate |
| 28 | 82.4 | Ventricular fibrillation possible |
| 27 | 80.6 | Loss of voluntary motion |
| **SEVERE** | | |
| 26 | 78.8 | Unresponsive to pain |
| 24 | 75.2 | Significant hypotension |
| 22 | 71.6 | Ventricular fibrillation likely |

Modified from Danze DF: Accidental hypothermia. In Rosen P (ed): Emergency Medicine: Concepts and Clinical Practice, 2nd ed. St Louis: CV Mosby, 1988, p. 667.

preexisting disease such as congestive heart failure can cause hypovolemia even at 70° F.

The following questions may be helpful in treating a person with hypothermia:

- What happened? If trauma has occurred, coexisting shock may compromise compensatory mechanisms and complicate treatment.

- How long has the patient been exposed to the cold?
  - —Hypothermia over a period of hours or days can occur in the elderly, especially in conjunction with alcohol, preexisting disease, malnutrition, hypoglycemia, and elder abuse or neglect.
  - —Cold water immersion can cause hypothermia after only a few minutes, but exposure to cold air at the same temperature takes longer to cause hypothermia.

### Assessment

1. Shivering stops at 88° F (31° C).

NOTE: Hypothermia resembles rigor mortis. People aren't dead until they are warm and dead.

2. Greatest risk is from ventricular fibrillation. Avoid rough handling, stimulation of the gag reflex, overventilation, unnecessary cardiac compressions, and active external rewarming.
3. Check for breathing with a mirror, if available.
4. Check pulse for a full minute.

### Treatment

1. Treatment is determined by the time it will take to transport the patient and the degree of hypothermia. Goals are to reduce further heat loss and to transport the patient rapidly to a medical facility for gentle active rewarming.
2. Reduce further heat loss by protecting the patient from wind. Remove wet clothes and provide blankets, sleeping bags, etc.
3. Carefully insert necessary airway device, and avoid stimulating the gag reflex.

## TABLE 4–2 ■ Wind Chill Chart

| Wind Speed | | Cooling Power of Wind Expressed as Equivalent Chill Temperature | | | | | | |
|---|---|---|---|---|---|---|---|---|
| Knots | Mph | Temperature (° F) | | | | | | |
| Calm | Calm | 25 | 20 | 15 | 10 | 5 | 0 | −5 |
| **EQUIVALENT CHILL TEMPERATURE** | | | | | | | | |
| 3–6 | 5 | 20 | 15 | 10 | 5 | 0 | −5 | −10 |
| 7–10 | 10 | 10 | 5 | 0 | −10 | −15 | −20 | −25 |
| 11–15 | 15 | 0 | −5 | −10 | −20 | −25 | −30 | −40 |
| 16–19 | 20 | 0 | −10 | −15 | −25 | −30 | −35 | −45 |
| 20–23 | 25 | −5 | −15 | −20 | −30 | −35 | −45 | −50 |
| 24–28 | 30 | −10 | −20 | −25 | −30 | −40 | −50 | −55 |
| 29–32 | 35 | −10 | −20 | −30 | −35 | −40 | −50 | −60 |
| 33–36 | 40 | −15 | −20 | −30 | −35 | −45 | −55 | −60 |
| Winds above 40 mph have little additional effect | | Little danger | | Increasing danger (flesh may freeze within 1 minute) | | | | |
| Danger of Freezing Exposed Flesh for Properly Clothed Persons | | | | | | | | |

Modified from the United States Air Force Survival Manual 64-3.

**Cooling Power of Wind Expressed as Equivalent Chill Temperature**

| Temperature (° F) | | | | | | | |
|---|---|---|---|---|---|---|---|
| −10 | −15 | −20 | −25 | −30 | −35 | −40 | −45 |
| −15 | −20 | −25 | −30 | −35 | −40 | −45 | −50 |
| −35 | −40 | −45 | −50 | −60 | −65 | −70 | −75 |
| −45 | −50 | −60 | −65 | −70 | −80 | −85 | −90 |
| −50 | −60 | −65 | −75 | −80 | −85 | −95 | −100 |
| −60 | −65 | −75 | −80 | −90 | −95 | −105 | −110 |
| −65 | −70 | −80 | −85 | −95 | −100 | −110 | −115 |
| −65 | −75 | −80 | −90 | −100 | −105 | −115 | −120 |
| −70 | −75 | −85 | −95 | −100 | −110 | −115 | −125 |

Great danger (flesh may freeze within 30 seconds)

Danger of Freezing Exposed Flesh for Properly Clothed Persons

4. Provide warm, humidified oxygen (50 percent concentration). If respiratory assistance is needed, *do not hyperventilate.*
5. If the patient is verbally responsive and has an intact gag reflex, give warm fluids containing sugar during a long transport.

NOTE: Do not give alcoholic or caffeinated beverages.

6. If the patient is unresponsive, be extremely careful when palpating for a pulse. Assess the pulse for one full minute.

NOTE: Cardiac compressions may have the adverse effect of precipitating ventricular fibrillation.

7. Once cardiopulmonary resuscitation is begun, it should be continued until relieved at the hospital or the pulse returns.

## Frostbite

Frostbite most often occurs to exposed areas of the skin: ears, nose, chin, cheeks, wrists, and fingers. The tissue damage is from ice crystals that form in the frozen area. The duration of exposure and the texture and color of the skin may indicate the seriousness of the frostbite.

### *Assessment*

1. The frostbitten area is usually sharply differentiated from normal tissue. *Never rub or massage frostbitten parts.*
2. Upon rewarming, there is a marked flush to the skin. Mottled areas may appear along with swelling and blisters.

*Treatment—Rapid Rewarming**

1. Immerse the affected part into a basin of warm water large enough to accommodate the part without it touching the container sides.
2. Preheat and maintain the water temperature at about 40.6° C (105° F), and keep it between 37.8° C and 43.3° C. If no thermometer is available, the water should cause only slight discomfort to normal skin. Water above 44° C is uncomfortable to most people.
3. Continuously stir the water to maintain a uniform temperature.
4. Most patients will feel pain on rethawing. The rewarming process is complete when the part is soft again and color and sensation return.
5. After rewarming, dress the area with sterile dressings. Do not break any blisters. Place folded sterile dressings between the toes or fingers before covering a foot or hand.

NOTE: The thawed part must be protected from refreezing. The rapid rewarming process can take from 20 to 40 minutes.

## DIFFICULTY BREATHING

Difficulty breathing or shortness of breath is one of the most common dispatches for EMTs and may be caused by many conditions, including **asthma** and

*Modified from Bangs C, Hamlet MP: Hypothermia and cold injuries. In Auerbach PS, Geehr EC (eds): Management of Wilderness and Environmental Emergencies. New York: Macmillan, 1983.

**chronic obstructive pulmonary disease** (COPD). A good history helps differentiate the causes.

***History.*** Remember that COPD patients are prone to **pneumonia.** A worsening of COPD can be triggered by **cardiac problems,** or vice versa. Important questions to ask include:

- How long have you had this episode of difficulty breathing?
  - —Asthma, COPD, pneumonia, and cardiac problems usually last hours with no relief, although there are exceptions (especially pneumonia).
- What were you doing when this started?
  - —Spontaneous pneumothorax and hyperventilation syndrome tend to be sudden and associated with an activity.
- Does anything make it worse?
  - —Lying down usually aggravates difficulty breathing from cardiac problems and sometimes pneumonia.
- Do you have any other complaints?
  - —Chest pain and dizziness are common with cardiac problems.
  - —Fever and productive cough is common with pneumonia. Elderly patients with pneumonia may not run a fever.
  - —A sharp pain at the onset of difficulty breathing or on inspiration is pleuritic and may indicate a spontaneous **pneumothorax.**
  - —Hyperventilation syndrome also may cause sharp chest pain after the episode has begun.
- What has changed?
  - —A change in productive cough from white **spu-**

**tum** to yellow, green, or gray indicates a probable infection.
  —A productive cough with white or pink foamy sputum is probably from cardiac-related pulmonary edema.
- Are you taking any medications?
  —Patients with cardiac problems often take "heart pills" (e.g., digoxin [Lanoxin] or digitalis), "blood pressure pills" (antihypertensives, e.g., propranolol [Inderal] or hydrochlorothiazide [Esidrex]), "water pills" (diuretics, e.g., furosemide [Lasix]), vasodilators (e.g., nitroglycerin [Nitro-Bid]), and calcium channel blockers (e.g., verapamil [Calan]).
  —Patients with COPD or asthma are often prescribed theophylline (Theo-Dur), isoetharine (Bronkosol), metaproterenol sulfate (Alupent), albuterol (Ventolin), oxtriphylline (Choledyl), and prednisone.

### *Assessment**

1. Ask about onset and history.
2. Note use of accessory breathing muscles or obvious respiratory compromise (such as inability to speak in complete sentences).
3. Evaluate need for ALS assistance. If not available, provide rapid transport.
4. Asthma and spontaneous **pneumothorax** generally occur in younger patients. However, older COPD patients often have blebs (fragile blisters)

*Modified from New York City Emergency Medical Services, Basic Life Support Protocols, 1990.

on their lungs that predispose them to spontaneous pneumothorax.

5. Early **pulmonary edema** presents with diminished lung sounds and wheezes. Check for **pitting edema,** which suggests pulmonary edema in the older patient.
6. Hyperventilation is usually a compensatory mechanism in difficulty breathing, except **hyperventilation** caused by an emotional event. If a hyperventilating patient without trauma cannot be talked down, suspect another cause, e.g., pulmonary embolism.
7. If patient has high-grade fever, muffled voice, inability to swallow, drooling, or describes pain as "worse sore throat in my life," suspect epiglottitis. Adults will spit instead of drool.
8. If patient has low-grade fever, a barking cough, and sternal retractions, suspect croup.

### *Treatment**

1. Maintain ABCs.
2. Administer high-concentration oxygen via mask nonrebreather or bag-valve-mask.
3. Reassure the patient and remain calm.
4. Do not permit physical exertion.
5. Monitor the patient's condition and document vital signs *every five minutes.*
6. Allow the patient to assume a comfortable position. A child may want to be held by the parent, *preferably in an upright position.*
7. Transport the patient to the hospital. Record all

*Modified from New York City Emergency Medical Services, Basic Life Support Protocols, 1990.

information, including medical history and all treatment provided.

***Special Precautions*.*** Be prepared to deal with respiratory and cardiac arrest! Monitor the respiratory status continuously. If the patient demonstrates inadequate ventilations (respiratory rate of more than 10 per minute or more than 29 per minute) and is confused, restless, or cyanotic, use the bag-valve-mask with reservoir or positive-pressure adjunctive breathing device.

## DROWNING (Near)

The typical victim has probably overestimated his or her endurance, is intoxicated, cannot swim, suffered a seizure, or has experienced trauma.

### *History**

1. Was diving or a fall involved? If spinal injuries are likely, a floatable backboard or similar device is necessary for removal. Remember, rescue breathing starts in the water.
2. Did the accident occur in fresh or salt water? The effects of fresh or salt water in the lungs vary.
3. About how long was the person submerged? What is the approximate water temperature? Both variables affect survivability.
4. Does the person have any medical problems that also may require treatment?

*Modified from New York City Emergency Medical Services, Basic Life Support Protocols, 1990.

5. If the patient is conscious at the scene but has a history of losing consciousness, he or she must be checked by a physician. Respiratory distress can occur hours after the incident.

### *Assessment**

1. If the victim is submerged when you arrive, request the scuba search and rescue unit to respond. Anticipate any necessary medical treatment and prepare all equipment accordingly.

NOTE: Rescues should not be attempted by those not properly trained in water rescue techniques.

### *Treatment*

1. Perform expanded primary survey, and begin artificial respiration if needed.
2. Remove the patient from the water, using spinal precautions as indicated. Treat for hypothermia if water temperature is below 70° F.
3. Transport, keeping the patient warm.

NOTE: In cold water, cerebral oxygen requirements are greatly reduced. These patients often can withstand cardiac arrest (even though submerged) for long periods of time without subsequent brain damage. Therefore, *always initiate and maintain resuscitation procedures when indicated.*

## HEAT EXPOSURE

The three types of heat exposure illnesses range in severity from heat cramps to heat exhaustion and

*Modified from New York City Emergency Medical Services, Basic Life Support Protocols, 1990.

heatstroke (Table 4–3). Figure 4–2 shows body temperatures for different conditions. (Fig. 4–3 shows the range of normal body temperatures.)

***History.*** The very young and elderly are most susceptible to heat-related illnesses. Also, many drugs (tranquilizers, antidepressants, amphetamines, diuretics, and antihistamines) lower a person's tolerance to heat. People using alcohol or cocaine as well as those who exercise excessively on hot humid days are particularly vulnerable.

NOTE: Heatstroke usually does not present with sweating. However, if the patient has been rigorously exercising, sweat may be present.

### *Treatment*

1. Remove the patient from the hot environment.
2. Assure airway control, administer oxygen as needed.
3. *If level of consciousness is intact:*
   - Gently stretch the cramped muscles and administer a weak saline solution (¼ teaspoon salt in quart of water), if available.
   - Loosen or remove clothing, apply fan or wet towels, and administer weak saline solution, if available, for weakness, exhaustion, or headache.
4. *If level of consciousness is altered:*
   - Apply cold packs to armpits, groin, and neck. Moisten sheets or towels with cool water, circulate air by fan, and turn up air-conditioner.
   - Apply high-concentration oxygen.

**TABLE 4–3 ■ Heat Emergencies**

| Condition | Signs and Symptoms | Treatment |
|---|---|---|
| Heat cramps | Muscular cramps following exercise | Cool environment<br>Fluid replacement with balanced saline solution<br>Stretch affected muscle |
| Heat exhaustion | Weakness or exhaustion<br>Dizziness, faintness<br>Skin moist, pale (or pink), may be cool<br>Vital signs normal or tachycardia, orthostatic hypotension, elevated temperature (<39° C) | Cooling efforts<br>Cool environment<br>Fanning<br>Loosen or remove clothing<br>Fluids<br>Supine position (legs elevated) |
| Heatstroke | Altered mental state<br>Hot, dry skin (may be moist)<br>Elevated body temperature (usually >40° C) | Aggressive cooling measures (wet sheets, fanning, ice to vessels of neck, armpits, groin)<br>Rapid transport<br>Oxygen |

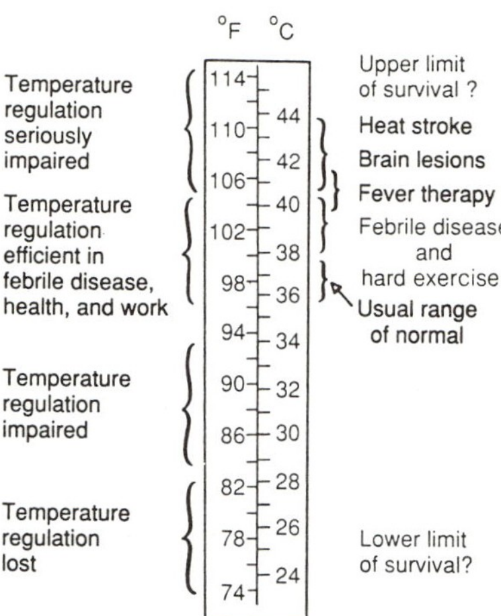


**Figure 4–2** Body temperatures under different conditions. (From Dubois, Fever and the Regulation of Body Temperature. Courtesy of Charles C Thomas, Publisher, Springfield, Illinois.)

- Record initial vital signs and repeat as often as necessary en route (every 5 to 15 minutes).
- Record all patient care information, including the medical history and all treatment provided on a prehospital care report.

## OBSTRUCTED AIRWAY

In adults, obstructed airways usually occur during a meal. Patients often are found in the restaurant restrooms. Usually a sudden collapse while eating

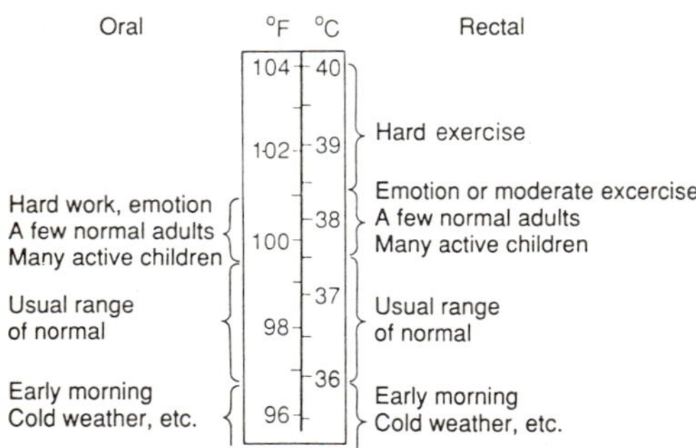


**Figure 4–3** Range of normal temperatures in humans. (From Dubois, Fever and the Regulation of Body Temperature. Courtesy of Charles C Thomas, Publisher, Springfield, Illinois.)

or a sudden departure from the table has occurred. For an obstructed airway in a child, see page 64.

### *History*

1. What was the patient doing when this happened? The most common cause is food ingested with alcohol while talking or laughing.
2. Was the patient complaining of anything before the incident? Chest pain or discomfort suggests a cardiac problem.

### *Assessment*

1. If the patient is unconscious, compare the rise and fall of the chest and stomach, which helps to determine if an obstruction is present.
2. Be prepared for vomiting, especially if abdominal thrusts are used.

3. Flushing, blotchy skin, or swollen eyes and tongue indicate an allergic reaction.

### *Treatment**

1. If the patient is conscious and can breathe, cough, or speak, do not interfere (i.e., encourage coughing).
2. If the foreign body cannot be dislodged by the patient coughing:
   - Administer high-concentration oxygen.
   - Transport in a sitting position, keeping the patient warm.
   - Obtain and record the vital signs, and repeat en route as often as necessary (at least every 15 minutes).
3. If the patient is conscious but cannot breathe, cough, or speak, or if the patient is or becomes unconscious, perform obstructed airway maneuvers according to AHA/ARC standards.

NOTE: If the obstructed airway is caused by trauma, manually immobilize the head and cervical spine in a neutral position while opening the patient's airway using the jaw-thrust maneuver, and transport the patient without delay!

4. If airway obstruction persists after two sequences of obstructed airway maneuvers
   - Transport, keeping the patient warm.
   - Repeat the sequences of obstructed airway ma-

*Modified from Manual for Emergency Medical Technicians. Emergency Medical Services Program. Albany: New York State Department of Health, 1990.

neuvers en route until the foreign body is forced out.
- Obtain and record the vital signs, and repeat en route as often as necessary (at least every 15 minutes).

5. If the airway obstruction is reversed and the patient resumes breathing:
   - Administer high-concentration oxygen.
   - Transport, keeping the patient warm.
   - Obtain and record the vital signs, and repeat en route as often as necessary (at least every 15 minutes).
6. Record all patient care information, including the patient's medical history and all treatment provided, on a Prehospital Care Report.

## POISONING AND DRUG OVERDOSE*

### *Assessment*

1. Survey the scene for any hazardous situations before entering. Drug overdose is a common method of suicide.
2. Look for remnants and containers of the poison or drug, drug paraphernalia, and vomitus. If possible, bring the substance and container with the patient to the hospital.
3. Determine the age and weight of the patient.
4. Attempt to determine the drug or poison by ask-

*Data from Manual for Emergency Medical Technicians. Emergency Medical Services Program. Albany: New York State Department of Health, 1990; and New York City EMS Academy Training Protocols.

ing: How was the substance taken and how much? How long ago was it taken? Was it taken all at once or over a period of time? Did the patient vomit? Were any antidotes taken? Was Poison Control contacted?

5. Determine the patient's present signs and symptoms, including hives (urticaria), injection sites, skin color, breath odor, and burns to mouth.
6. Determine the patient's medical history:
   - Does the patient work with fertilizers, insecticides, or other hazardous chemicals? Look for containers.
   - If the patient was at a party, consider drug overdose.
   - The presence of track or needle marks increases the likelihood of communicable diseases; use precautions.
7. If the patient is unconscious, maintain ABCs, determine GCS score (see pages 42–43), and record the findings.
8. If alcohol is involved, prepare to assist ventilation and anticipate vomiting. Alcohol has a potentiating affect on many street drugs.
9. Assess the need for ALS. Remember that ALS is often helpful in poisonings such as narcotics and insecticides.

### Treatment

*For conscious patients*

1. Remove the patient from any hazards.
2. Maintain ABCs.
3. Administer high-concentration oxygen.
4. Assist ventilations as necessary by bag-valve-

mask with supplemental oxygen or demand valve resuscitator.

NOTE: These patients may deteriorate rapidly. Be especially alert for respiratory insufficiency or arrest.

5. Provide rapid transport if history and assessment dictate.

*For unconscious patients*

1. Assure that the patient's airway is open and that breathing and circulation are adequate; suction as necessary.
2. Administer high-concentration oxygen.
3. Provide rapid transport, keeping the patient warm.
4. Obtain and record the vital signs, and repeat as necessary en route to the hospital.
5. Record all patient care information, including the patient's medical history and all treatment provided, on the prehospital care report.

*For swallowed poisons*

1. If possible, contact the Poison Control Center or EMS Telemetry Control for instructions on treatment, which may include the administration of milk, water, or ipecac syrup (to cause vomiting). **Caution:** Do not induce vomiting when hydrocarbons, acids and bases, or caustic substances have been ingested.
2. Maintain ABCs.
3. Provide rapid transport, keeping the patient warm.
4. Obtain and record the vital signs and repeat as necessary.
5. Special precautions:
   a. Do not attempt to neutralize poisons or drugs

or to induce vomiting unless directed to do so by Poison Control or EMS radio control.

b. Dilution of poisons or induction of vomiting is contraindicated in unconscious or convulsive patients.

*Inhaled poisons*

1. Assure that the scene is safe for entry. If poisonous gases, vapors, or sprays or a low-oxygen environment is present, it may be necessary to obtain assistance from trained rescue personnel with self-contained breathing apparatus (SCBA).
2. Remove the patient to an area with fresh air.
3. Place the patient in a comfortable position.
4. Ensure that the patient's airway is open and that breathing and circulation are adequate.
5. Administer high-concentration oxygen.
6. Provide rapid transport, keeping the patient warm.
7. Obtain and record vital signs, and repeat as necessary en route.

*For injected substances*

1. Attempt to calm the patient.
2. Remove jewelry from the affected area if swelling begins.
3. Place the injection site lower than the patient's heart, if possible.
4. If the injury is from a reptile, implement snakebite procedures (see page 132).

*Surface contact substances*

1. Remove patient from source (e.g., Mace, lye, or industrial chemicals) as soon as this can be done *safely*.
2. Remove all contaminated clothing.

3. Rinse affected area thoroughly with saline solution or sterile or plain water for 20 minutes. **Caution:** Some chemicals are more harmful with water, such as dry lime and calcium metal.
4. Maintain ABCs.
5. Bandage any substance burns with a dry sterile dressing. See also Eye Injuries, pages 148–149.

## RAPE OR SEXUAL ASSAULT

### *Special Considerations*

1. Preserve the patient's privacy as much as possible. Clear away bystanders.
2. Ask the victim to come to the hospital for proper examination, treatment, and preservation of evidence. Advise the patient not to urinate, defecate, wash, shower, brush teeth, or douche before being examined because evidence may be destroyed. If clothing has been changed, bring the old clothes to the hospital in a paper sack.
3. Perform a complete assessment; treat wounds accordingly. If the patient evaluation and treatment take place at the crime scene, interfere as little as possible, being careful not to litter unnecessarily with dressing wrappers and other materials.
4. Patient may reject treatment by a male EMT. If a woman EMT is available, she should take over care. If not, do as the situation dictates.
5. Impaled objects in the urethra, vagina, or rectum should be treated as you would other impaled injuries, with the object left in place to tamponade possible internal bleeding until it can be removed at the hospital.

6. If the patient refuses care, respect his or her wishes. In rape or sexual assault cases, it is important to leave the patient with a friend or other person who can offer comfort and support. It also is important to give the victim the contact number for the local rape counseling center.

### *Legal Concerns*

1. Questions should be medically related and directed to obtain information to treat the patient. Do not ask questions about the assault beyond what is needed to care for the patient. A detailed history can be taken at the hospital.
2. If the patient recounts events of the assault, record the statements just as they are given (e.g., "Patient states, 'I was raped . . .'"). Be precise. Your record will probably be scrutinized if the patient presses charges, and you may be called to testify in court. Remember, your job is that of a medical professional; you are not a legal authority or police officer.
3. Clothing discarded at the scene should be collected and placed in a bag with as little handling as possible since it may contain semen, blood, hairs, or other evidence that may help identify the rapist. If clothing must be removed to treat injuries, save in a paper bag and keep it in your presence until hand-delivered to hospital staff or a police officer.
4. Maintain a chain of custody for any evidence,

including clothing, by recording what happened to any belongings, to whom you delivered them, and when. They should co-sign the patient record beside your notation.

## SEIZURES

The causes of seizures include epilepsy, head injury, rapid rise in temperature, hypoxia, hypoglycemia, infections, drug overdose, and drug withdrawal. Grand mal seizures are the type most often seen by EMTs. Ask the following questions:

- Has this happened before? Do they have a history of seizures? If not, assess the possible cause while preparing the patient for transport to the hospital.
- Has the patient run a fever, been hit on the head, had a recent infection, or been acting unusual? Bruises indicate trauma, but if bruising is of similar shape, size, and color all over the body, suspect systemic infection.
- Has the patient taken any medications today? If so, was the normal amount taken?
- Does the patient have any medical problems?
  - — If diabetic, suspect diabetic reaction, especially if the breath smells of acetone (overripe fruit).
  - — If epileptic, ask if they have taken their medications.
  - — If unequal pupils, suspect intracranial hemorrhage.

### *Treatment for Patient Who Is Seizing**

1. Protect the patient from harm by removing hazards from the immediate area, and avoid unnecessary physical restraint.
2. Ensure that the patient's airway is open. **Caution:** *Never force the patient's mouth open or force an oral airway or other device into the mouth if it is clenched tightly during the seizure!* A nasal airway may be used instead. Turn patient on side to aid drainage of secretions.
3. Suction the airway as needed. Avoid stimulation of the posterior pharynx during suctioning because this may cause vomiting.
4. Administer high-concentration oxygen and ventilate, if needed.
5. Transport immediately, keeping the patient warm.
6. Obtain and record the vital signs, and report en route as necessary.
7. Record all patient care information, including the medical history and all treatment provided, on the prehospital care report.

### *Treatment for Postseizure Patient**

1. Ensure that the patient's airway is open and that breathing and circulation are adequate.
2. Administer high-concentration oxygen.
3. Treat any injuries sustained during the seizure.
4. Be prepared for additional seizures.

*Modified from Manual for Emergency Medical Technicians. Emergency Medical Services Program. Albany: New York State Department of Health, 1990.

5. Obtain and record the vital signs, and repeat en route, as necessary.
6. If the patient regains consciousness, orient to surroundings.

## SNAKEBITES

Snake venom is either necrotoxic (causing local necrosis) or neurotoxic (causing systemic effects) or both. The treatment and antidote differ depending on the type of venom. If the snake has been killed, bring it along with the patient.

### *Treatment*

1. Keep the patient calm, and immobilize the extremity with a splint.
2. If swelling is present, make a small mark with a pen at its edge so any changes are evident on later evaluation.
3. Transport the victim to the nearest hospital capable of caring for snakebites.

### *Special Precautions*

1. Follow local protocols for coral snakebite (e.g., applying a pressure bandage over the bite to decrease systemic absorption). Be sure you know your local protocols for treating snakebite.
2. For any type of snakebite, do not use ice or cut the wound and attempt to suck out the venom.

## STROKE

In a stroke, or cerebrovascular accident (CVA), vessels rupture or become blocked, which disrupts blood flow to the brain. Signs and symptoms depend on the area affected. A history of high blood pressure is the most common predictor, but persons of any age, regardless of history, can have a stroke.

- Nausea, vomiting, seizures, and incontinence are commonly associated with stroke.
- One-sided sensory loss and motor weakness are immediate signs of strokes.
- In patients who have been drinking, remember that strokes mimic intoxication.
- Even though the patient may not be able to respond, he or she may still understand you. *Always assume the patient can understand you.*
- A headache with sudden onset that gets increasingly worse suggests an intracerebral bleed.

### Assessment*

1. Determine GCS score (see pages 42–43) and record all findings.
2. Document any neurologic deficits.
3. Note medical history—especially diabetes and hypertension.

### Treatment*

1. Maintain ABCs and intervene as required.
2. Administer high-concentration oxygen.
3. Place the patient in a semi-sitting position, if he or she is conscious. If unconscious, transport the patient in the coma position.
4. *Do not permit physical activity!*

*Modified from Basic Life Support Protocols. New York City Emergency Medical Services, 1990.

5. Monitor the patient's condition and document vital signs as indicated.
6. Transport the patient to the appropriate hospital.

## SUICIDE (Attempted)

Psychoanalysts theorize that depression is caused by anger being turned inward, which in extreme cases, can result in suicide (i.e., aggression against self). However, aggression turned inward can easily be turned toward others, even those trying to help. Remember that your safety comes first; call law enforcement as soon as an attempted suicide is suspected.

### *Special Concerns*

1. Try to find out if the patient has been on any medication and if it has been taken.
2. If there is any doubt, ask the patient if they have thought of suicide. Ask how it was planned, then remove the means for carrying it out, if present. Also remove any harmful objects from the vicinity of the patient.
3. Do not leave the patient alone at any time.
4. Bring any pills, containers, or other materials that may assist in patient diagnosis or treatment to the hospital.
5. If appropriate, have police accompany the patient in the ambulance.

***Treatment.*** Treatment is symptomatic

# TRAUMA

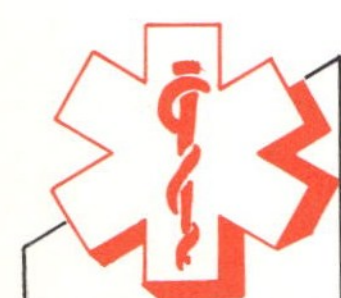

## MAJOR TRAUMA (Including Traumatic Cardiac Arrest)

The protocol for major trauma, including traumatic cardiac arrest, in adults is given on page 136. For trauma in children, see pages 72–74. Not all patients with major injury present with abnormal assessments. In these cases, the mechanism of injury should be the guide for determining the potential seriousness of the victim. Such patients should then be transported to the appropriate hospital. Often the only indication of potential seriousness is the level of anxiety of the patient and prevailing "sense of doom" that cannot be calmed. Remember, the presence of unreasonable anxiety in the patient usually indicates the presence of a potentially lethal injury.

## PROTOCOL
## Major Trauma (Including Traumatic Cardiac Arrest)

### Definition

For the purpose of this protocol, major trauma is present if the mechanism of injury or patient's physical findings meets *any one* of the following criteria (see pages 33–35).

### Mechanism of Injury

1 Fall of two or more stories (more than 20 feet)
2 Survivor of motor vehicle crash in which there was a death of a car occupant
3 Patient struck by a vehicle moving faster than 20 mph
4 Patient ejected from the vehicle
5 High-speed crash with resulting severe deformity of the vehicle
6 Rollover

### Physical Findings

7 Pulse less than 50/minute or greater than 120/minute
8 Systolic blood pressure of 90 mm Hg or less
9 Respiratory rate less than 10/minute or greater than 28/minute
10 GCS score less than 13
11 All penetrating injuries of the trunk, head, neck, chest, abdomen, or groin
12 Two or more proximal long bone fractures

13 Flail chest
14 Burns that involve 15 percent or more of the body surface or facial/airway burns

**Procedure**

1 Establish and maintain airway control while manually stabilizing the cervical spine.
*The following management may be instituted before or during extrication or en route as appropriate. In no case should patient transport be delayed because of this management!*

2 Assess the patient's ventilatory status.
  **a** *If the ventilatory status is inadequate:*
    **(1)** Insert an oropharyngeal or nasopharyngeal airway if the gag reflex is absent.
    **(2)** Ventilate the patient with an adjunctive device and high-concentration oxygen. *Minimum rate of ventilation: 12 times a minute. Make certain that the chest rises with each ventilation.*

**AND**

*Expose the patient's chest to locate and identify injuries and to listen for breath sounds.*

**AND**

*Treat any open chest wounds with oc-*

*Continued.*

*clusive dressing, and stabilize impaled objects in the chest.*

b *If the ventilatory status is adequate* administer high-concentration oxygen as soon as possible.

c *If head injury is suspected, hyperventilate the patient with high-concentration oxygen at a rate of about 20 breaths per minute!*

3 Assess the patient's circulatory status.

a *If the pulse is absent (traumatic cardiac arrest):*

(1) Extricate the patient rapidly.

(2) Initiate transportation *immediately*.

(3) Perform CPR according to AHA/ARC standards.

(4) Take appropriate steps to control hemorrhage.

(5) Apply and inflate MAST according to the

(a) Shock Protocol, *OR*

(b) Elevate the patient's legs 30 degrees if MAST are not available.

(6) Record all patient care information, including all treatment provided, on a prehospital care report.

b *If the pulse is present:*

(1) Search for any life-threatening hemorrhage and test capillary refill.

(2) Extricate the patient rapidly.

(3) Initiate transportation *immediately*.

(4) Keep the patient warm en route.

(5) Obtain and record the initial vital signs, including capillary refill, and repeat en route as often as the situation indicates.

(6) Record all patient care information, including all treatment provided, on a prehospital care report.

**c** *If life-threatening hemorrhage is present:*

(1) Take appropriate steps to control the hemorrhage.

(2) Extricate the patient rapidly.

(3) Initiate transportation *immediately*.

(4) Keep the patient warm en route.

(5) Assess for *shock* en route.

(6) Obtain and record the initial vital signs, including capillary refill, and repeat en route as often as the situation indicates.

(7) Record all patient care information, including all treatment provided, on a prehospital care report.

**d** *If one or more signs of shock are present, refer immediately to the Shock Protocol*

(1) Extricate the patient rapidly.

(2) Initiate transportation *immediately*.

(3) Apply and inflate MAST according to the

(a) Shock Protocol *OR*

*Continued.*

(b) Elevate the patient's legs 30 degrees if MAST are not available.

(4) Keep the patient warm.

(5) Obtain and record the initial vital signs, including capillary refill, and repeat en route as often as the situation indicates.

(6) Record all patient care information, including all treatment provided, on a prehospital care report. ■

From Manual for Emergency Medical Technicians. Emergency Medical Services Program. Albany: New York State Department of Health, 1990.

## ABDOMINAL TRAUMA

1. *Treat the whole patient.* In the setting of multiple blunt trauma, immobilize the spine, and treat life-threatening injuries.
2. *Maintain the airway,* especially in the presence of vomiting. Patients with altered mental status and vomiting should be positioned in the left lateral recumbent position, with suction on standby to aid in keeping the airway clear en route. For patients who are immobilized on a spine board, be aware that the patient may have to be turned as a unit if vomiting occurs. Suction must be available.
3. *Give high-concentration oxygen* if shock or internal bleeding is present.

4. *Control external bleeding,* secure penetrating objects in place, and dress open wounds.
5. *Treat for shock* if present. Maintain body temperature, elevate legs, and consider using MAST.
6. *Position the patient* according to the need for spinal immobilization, airway maintenance, positive-pressure breathing, shock treatment, and comfort. Patients with abdominal injuries may find the most comfort from being transported supine, with hips and knees flexed. A pillow may be placed under the knees.
7. *Give nothing by mouth.* The patient with an abdominal emergency may require surgery.
8. *Complete the examination en route* to the hospital. Repeat vital signs as indicated. Record your findings.
9. *Select the hospital* by local protocols for trauma center candidates. Notify the hospital of the impending arrival.

## BURNS

The treatment for burns is the same whether they are caused by electrical or thermal sources. Burns are classified according to depth (Table 5–1). It is important to estimate the area of the burn in relation to the total body surface by using the rule of nines (Fig. 5–1). For smaller area burns, the palm of the patient's hand is usually equivalent to about 1 percent of the patient's body surface area.

## TABLE 5–1 ■ Clinical Classification of Burn Depth

| | | Second-Degree (Partial Thickness) |
|---|---|---|
| | First-Degree | Superficial |
| Color | Bright red | Red and mottled |
| Surface | Dry with focal exfoliation | Blisters with copious exudate |
| Sensation | Painful | Painful |
| Time for healing | 3–6 days | 10–21 days |
| Cause | Sun or minor flash injury | Flash injury; spill scalds |

From American College of Surgeons: Early Care of the Injured Patient, 3rd ed. Philadelphia: WB Saunders, 1982, p. 88.

| Second-Degree (Partial Thickness) | |
|---|---|
| **Deep** | **Third-Degree (Full Thickness)** |
| Dark red or pale yellow to off-white | Very dark red in children; pearly white, charred; translucent and parchmentlike. Bronzed—strong acid injury; dissolution of skin with exposed deep tissues—strong alkali injury |
| Denuded surface with minimal exudate | Dry and leathery with thrombosed dermal and subdermal vessels visible. Smooth and silky—strong acid injury; liquefaction necrosis—strong alkali injury |
| Diminished pinprick sensation; intact dermal sensation | Anesthetic except for deep pressure sensation in subdermal tissues |
| More than 3 weeks | Grafting always required |
| Scalds of longer duration; flash of high intensity; brief exposure to flame | Flame burns; strong chemicals; contact with hot objects; electricity; prolonged scalds |

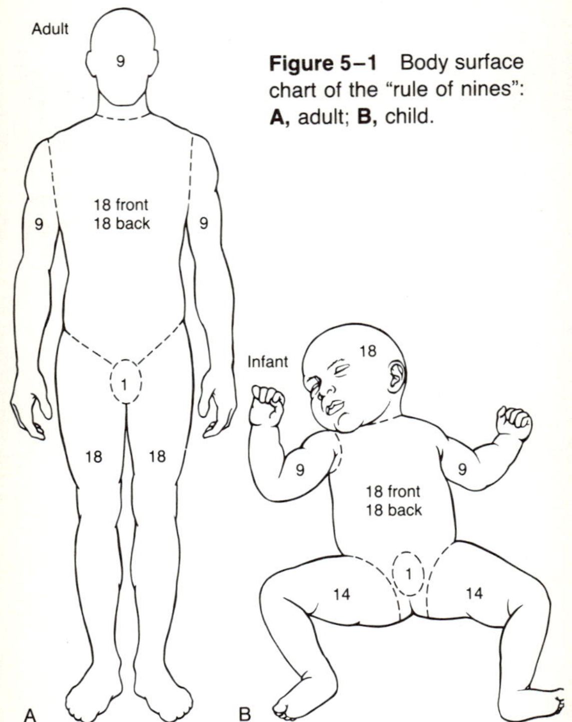


**Figure 5–1** Body surface chart of the "rule of nines": **A,** adult; **B,** child.

## *Treatment**

1. Assure that the scene is safe for entry. If not, obtain assistance from trained firefighters.

*Modified from Manual for Emergency Medical Technicians. Emergency Medical Services Program. Albany: New York State Department of Health, 1990.

2. Extinguish burning clothing, and stop the burning process. **Caution:** Manually stabilize the head and cervical spine if trauma to the head and neck is suspected.
3. Ensure that the patient's airway is open and that breathing and circulation are adequate.
4. Place the patient in a position of comfort only if doing so does not compromise stabilization of the head and cervical spine.
5. Administer high-concentration oxygen if respiratory burns are suspected and in all burns involving flames.
6. Assess for shock. If present, refer to page 153.
7. Remove smoldering clothing not adhering to the patient and rings, bracelets, and other constricting items.
8. For all burns, apply dry sterile dressing to the burned area.

NOTE: Do not puncture unbroken blisters!

9. Obtain and record the initial vital signs, and repeat en route as often as necessary.
10. Transport, keeping the patient warm. Turn up the heater and use blankets over sterile dressing. **Caution:** Burn patients tend to lose heat and become hypothermic!

## CHEST INJURIES

### *Special Considerations**

1. Note any deformities or abnormalities of the chest wall, including puncture wounds, sucking

*Modified from New York City Emergency Medical Services: Basic Life Support Protocols, 1990.

chest wounds, flail chest (an unstable segment of the chest wall), and paradoxical or asymmetrical chest movement.

2. Note and correct any respiratory distress.
3. Note if the patient is coughing up bright red blood or pink froth.
4. Check for the presence of subcutaneous emphysema in the skin overlying the chest or in the neck.
5. Check for jugular vein distention or tracheal deviation.
6. Note if the systolic and diastolic blood pressures are approximating each other (pericardial tamponade).
7. Check for the presence and equality of lung sounds (pneumothorax or hemothorax).
8. The patient should be considered as having a developing tension pneumothorax if any of the following exists:
   - Increasing difficulty in breathing.
   - Absent or greatly diminished breath sounds on one side.
   - Neck vein distention.
   - Movement of the trachea away from the pneumothorax to the unaffected side.
   - Progressive development of shock.

## Treatment*

*In general*

1. Maintain ABCs.
2. Administer high-concentration oxygen.

*Modified from New York City Emergency Medical Services: Basic Life Support Protocols, 1990.

3. Assist respirations as necessary.

NOTE: Do not use a demand-valve resuscitator!

4. Control external bleeding, including placement of occlusive dressings as necessary.
5. Initiate appropriate subprotocols.
6. Treat for shock.
7. Monitor vital signs.
8. Position the patient appropriately.
9. Transport as soon as possible.

*For open (sucking) chest wounds*

1. Control external bleeding.
2. Seal wound with occlusive dressing (e.g., sterile Vaseline gauze, plastic, or aluminum foil), and tape on three sides. This forms a flutter valve to prevent tension pneumothorax.
3. Seal should be made on exhalation.
4. If tension pneumothorax develops, unseal one side of the dressing to relieve pressure and then reseal it during exhalation.
5. Position the patient on the affected side.

*For flail chest*

1. Place bulky dressings over the flail segment and tape or bind in place.
2. Position the patient on the affected side.

*For possible simple rib fractures*

1. Either bind the arm to the affected side with a sling and swathe *or* place bulky dressings over the injury site and bind with sling and swathe.
2. Allow the patient to assume a comfortable position.
3. Continue to assess for development of complications after chest trauma.

2. Retrieve any lost tissue and transport with patient.

## FRACTURES

### *Treatment*

1. Maintain an airway, especially in presence of vomiting.
2. Assess for shock, and if present, administer high-concentration oxygen (see pages 50–51).
3. Place the patient in a comfortable position provided that injuries, control of airway, or treatment for shock do not contraindicate this.
4. Check distal pulses, capillary return, skin color and temperature, sensation, and motor function.
5. Gently straighten angulated fracture unless extreme pain or resistance is encountered. First, stabilize the joint above the fracture. Next, gently pull the extremity in the direction of angulation to separate bone ends, then gently pull in the direction of the bone's long axis until aligned. *Do not forcefully attempt to straighten a locked extremity.*
6. Cover open wounds with sterile dressings.
7. Splint the fracture and adjacent joints.
8. Recheck distal pulses, capillary return, skin color and temperature, sensation, and motor function. *If neurovascular function is compromised, gently loosen the splint.* If neurovascular function does not return, transport rapidly.
9. Repeat and record vital signs en route as often as indicated.
10. Transport, keeping the patient warm.

## HEAD OR SPINAL INJURIES

Suspected head or spinal injuries that do not meet major trauma criteria are treated as follows.

### *Treatment**

1. Establish and maintain airway control while manually stabilizing the cervical spine.
2. Assess the patient's ventilatory status, and administer high-concentration oxygen. Suction and assist patient's ventilations as necessary.

NOTE: If head injury is suspected, the patient is not alert, the arms and legs are abnormally flexed and/or extended (neurologic posturing), or the patient is seizing or has a GCS score of less than 8 (see pages 42–43), hyperventilate the patient.

3. Assess the patient's circulatory status.
4. Obtain and record the initial vital signs, including the GCS score and a neurologic assessment, i.e., level of consciousness (AVPU) and pupils (see pages 42–43 and 46), and sensory and motor function in the extremities, before and after spinal immobilization.
5. Immobilize the patient's head and spine with a rigid cervical collar and an appropriate immobilization device, e.g., a Kendrick Extrication Device (KED), Kansas Board, XP1, or short board if the patient is sitting or a long board if the patient is in a face-up position.

*Modified from Manual for Emergency Medical Technicians. Emergency Medical Services Program. Albany: New York State Department of Health, 1990.

A low systolic blood pressure means that the shock is severe.

NOTE: If a cardiac cause for shock is suspected, refer immediately to the cardiac-related protocol!

**Procedure**

1 Ensure that the patient's airway is open and that breathing and circulation are adequate.

   a **CAUTION!: Manually stabilize the head and cervical spine if trauma of the head and neck is suspected!**

2 Administer high-concentration oxygen, and *be prepared to ventilate the patient!*

3 Place the patient in a face-up position.

   **and**

   Elevate the patient's legs 30 degrees.

   a *In adults, if available, apply MAST. If the systolic blood pressure is below 90 mm Hg and signs of inadequate perfusion are present,* inflate all three compartments at the maximum pressure (about 100 mm Hg) *or* until the pop-off valves of all three compartments pop open.

   b *In children,* if available, apply and inflate appropriate size MAST according to criteria for inflation. Inflate the leg compartments until the pop-off valves pop open. If MAST is used, assist ventilations with bag-valve-mask (BVM).

c *Do not delay patient transport to apply and inflate MAST!*

d CAUTION:

(1) **If the patient has pulmonary edema, do not inflate MAST!**

(2) **If the patient has an evisceration or an impaled object in the abdomen or legs, inflate only the MAST compartments not overlying the evisceration or impaled object!**

(3) **If the patient is known to be pregnant, inflate only the MAST leg compartments!**

**5** Obtain and record the vital signs, and repeat en route as often as the situation indicates.

**6** Transport, keeping the patient warm.

**7** Record all patient care information, including the patient's medical history and all treatment provided, on a Prehospital Care Report.

NOTE: Once inflated, MAST must not be deflated in the field without physician direction! ■

Modified from Manual for Emergency Medical Technicians. Emergency Medical Services Program. Albany: New York State Department of Health, 1990.

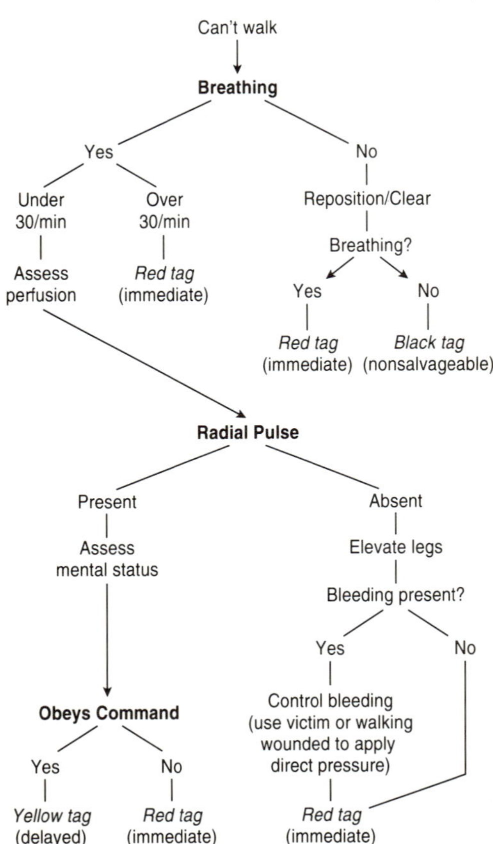
Ask those who can walk to move to a specific area → *Green tag* (hold)
Can't walk
**Breathing**
Yes
No
Under 30/min
Over 30/min
Assess perfusion
*Red tag* (immediate)
Reposition/Clear
Breathing?
Yes
No
*Red tag* (immediate)
*Black tag* (nonsalvageable)
**Radial Pulse**
Present
Absent
Assess mental status
Elevate legs
Bleeding present?
Yes
No
**Obeys Command**
Yes
No
Control bleeding (use victim or walking wounded to apply direct pressure)
*Yellow tag* (delayed)
*Red tag* (immediate)
*Red tag* (immediate)

**Figure 5–2** Algorithm for initial triage assessment. (From Cleary V, Hewett M, Schmehl A: START Instructor's Manual, 2nd ed.)

## TRIAGE

A triage system should be used whenever the number of patients exceeds the personnel who can give adequate care, as after an airplane crash. Mass casualties, as from a natural disaster, are beyond the scope of this handbook. However, EMTs may encounter five or more patients in car accidents, so triage is often necessary to assign treatment priorities and to make transport decisions.

Table 5–2 provides a color-coded priority system. Figure 5–2 shows an algorithm on performing rapid assessment based on Simple Triage and Rapid Transport (START), originally developed in California.

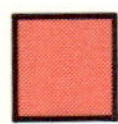

## APPENDIX B
## Inserting an Esophageal Gastric Tube Airway *Continued*

directly behind the trachea and result in a posterior collapse of the trachea.

- In persons with known esophageal disease or who have ingested caustic poisons. Here the integrity of the esophageal wall may be compromised, resulting in rupture.
- When there are facial injuries that prevent a tight seal with the mask.
- In conscious or breathing patients and patients who gag on insertion of the device.

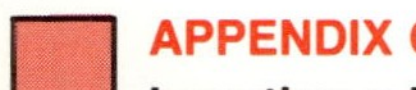

# APPENDIX C
## Inserting a Nasopharyngeal Airway

1. Lubricate the outside of the tube with a water-soluble gel to decrease irritation to the nasal passage.
2. Slowly insert the tube into either nasal passage. Do not force it in or nasal bleeding may occur, resulting in potential aspiration. Gentle, firm pressure sometimes results in dilation of one nasal passage and facilitates insertion.
3. If you are unable to successfully insert the tube in one nostril, you may try the opposite one.
4. Once inserted, test patency by initiating a ventilation and observing the chest rise while listening and feeling for air exchange.

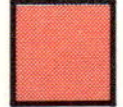

# APPENDIX E
## Metric Conversion Tables

### Liquid Measurements

| | | |
|---|---|---|
| 1 tsp = | 5 cc = | ⅙ oz |
| 1 tbsp = | 15 cc = | ½ oz |
| 2 tbsp = | 30 cc = | 1 oz |
| 1 cup = | 240 cc = | 8 oz |
| 1 pint = | 500 cc = | 16 oz |
| 1 quart = | 1000 cc = | 32 oz |

### Linear Measurements

| | |
|---|---|
| 1 millimeter (mm) | = 0.04 inch |
| 1 centimeter (cm) | = 0.4 inch |
| 2.5 centimeters | = 1 inch |
| 1 meter | = 39.37 inches |

### Weight Equivalents

| | |
|---|---|
| 1 oz = | 30 grams |
| 1 kg = | 1000 grams |
| 1 kg = | 2.2 lb |
| 1 lb = | 0.45 kg |

## Temperature Equivalents (°F)

| | | | |
|---|---|---|---|
| 98° (rectal) = | 97° (oral) = | 97° (forehead) = | 96° (axillary) |
| 99° (rectal) = | 98° (oral) = | 98° (forehead) = | 97° (axillary) |
| 100° (rectal) = | 99° (oral) = | 99° (forehead) = | 98° (axillary) |

*Rule of thumb:* rectal temperature 1° higher than an oral or forehead temperature; 2° higher than an axillary temperature

## Temperature

| Celsius<br>(C° × 9/5) + 32 = F° | Fahrenheit<br>(F° − 32) × 5/9 = C° |
|---|---|
| 0 | 32 |
| 35.0 | 96.8 |
| 36.5 | 97.7 |
| 37.0 | 98.6 |
| 37.5 | 99.5 |
| 38.0 | 100.4 |
| 38.5 | 101.3 |
| 39.0 | 102.2 |
| 39.5 | 103.1 |
| 40.0 | 104.0 |
| 40.5 | 104.9 |
| 41.0 | 105.8 |
| 41.5 | 106.7 |
| 42.0 | 107.6 |

From Damon SK, Graves JR: Patient Care Guidelines for the EMT. Englewood Cliffs, N.J.: Prentice-Hall, 1989, pp. 132–133.

*For suspected tension pneumothorax or pericardial tamponade*

1. Maintain ABCs.
2. Transport immediately if a tension pneumothorax is suspected.
3. En route to the appropriate hospital:
   a. Administer high-concentration oxygen.
   b. Treat other life-threatening injuries as necessary.
   c. With tension pneumothorax, position patient on the affected side unless contraindicated.
   d. Treat for shock.
   e. If ventilation assistance is required, place patient in the supine position, and assist ventilation by bag-valve-mask (*not* a demand-valve resuscitator) with supplemental oxygen.

*For traumatic asphyxia*

1. Maintain ABCs.
2. Control major external bleeding.
3. Administer high-concentration of oxygen.
4. Immobilize the patient's spine and stabilize the flail sternum.
5. Treat for shock.
6. If ventilation assistance is required, use modified jaw thrust and oropharyngeal airway to open the airway, and assist ventilation by bag-valve-mask (*not* a demand-valve resuscitator) with supplemental oxygen.

## EYE INJURIES

The eyes are very sensitive to injury. Improper handling may result in further damage and loss of vision. There are four important principles to remember:

1. Direct pressure must never be applied to an injured eyeball.
2. Cover *both* eyes to limit movement.
3. A chemical exposure to the eyes requires immediate, *continuous* irrigation (all the way to the hospital). If one eye is to be irrigated, do *not* allow runoff to flow into the other eye.
4. The patient's cooperation is needed when treating eye injuries. Explain your actions.

### *Removing a Foreign Object from the Eye*

1. Irrigation is the preferred method for removing foreign objects. Use sterile water or saline with an IV administration set or a specially packaged eye-irrigating solution.
2. Allow a gentle stream of water to pass from the medial portion of the sclera (part of eye closest to the nose) over the rest of the eyeball as you attempt to flush away the foreign body.
3. Respect the delicacy of the eyeball and *do not* use a high-pressure stream.
4. Rinse the affected portion of the eyelid, if necessary.

### *Impaled Object*

1. Stabilize object in place.
2. Be especially careful to cover both eyes.

### *Torn or Avulsed Eyelid*

1. Keep eye moist with moist sterile dressing.

6. Repeat and record the vital signs, including the GCS score and level of consciousness, en route as often as the situation indicates.
7. Transport, keeping the patient warm.

## INDUSTRIAL ACCIDENTS

Industrial accidents often involve patients entangled in machinery. Most companies have procedures for disabling equipment. Use company mechanics to disassemble machinery.

NOTE: Under no circumstances will the EMT work on a patient until the equipment has been turned off and disabled.

In some cases, it may be impossible to extricate the patient completely. If so, transport the patient with the equipment; this may require using other vehicles such as a flatbed truck. Do not remove impaled machinery.

## SHOCK

The protocol for shock in adults follows. For shock in children, see pages 69–74. The first sign of shock in children is usually manifested in an altered level of consciousness. Most children become lethargic and sleepy, although some may become combative. The heart rate becomes tachycardic, but the blood pressure is maintained until decompensation occurs. Peripheral vasoconstriction is obvious and very effective.

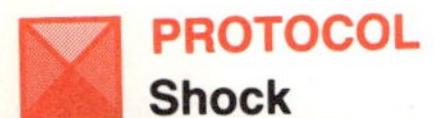

# PROTOCOL
## Shock

**Adult**

For the purpose of this protocol, adult shock is defined as:

1 Systolic blood pressure of 90 mm Hg or less
2 Systolic blood pressure above 90 mm Hg and signs of inadequate perfusion, such as:
   a Altered mental state (restlessness, inattention, confusion, agitation)
   b Tachycardia (pulse greater than 100)
   c Delayed capillary refill (greater than 2 seconds)
   d Pallor
   e Cold, clammy skin

**Pediatric**

For the purpose of this protocol, pediatric shock is defined as signs of inadequate perfusion such as:

1 Altered mental state (restlessness, inattention, confusion, agitation)
2 Tachycardia
3 Weak or absent distal pulses
4 Capillary refill greater than two seconds
5 Pallor
6 Cold, clammy, or mottled skin

*This protocol should be used even if the systolic blood pressure is normal or is difficult to obtain.*

Continued.

**TABLE 5–2 ■ Triage Protocol**

| Priority/Handling | Color Code |
| --- | --- |
| Immediate | Red |
| Delayed | Yellow |
| Hold | Green |
| Deceased | Black |

Modified from New York State Department of Health MCI Manual.

| Description | Patient Diagnosis |
|---|---|
| Life- or limb-threatening situations requiring immediate care | Airway or respiratory difficulties, severe burns, cardiac problems, uncontrollable or severe hemorrhage, open chest or abdominal wounds, severe head injury, severe medical problems, shock |
| Patients requiring care but will not worsen with delay | Burns, multiple or major fractures, spinal cord injuries, uncomplicated head injuries |
| Patients with minor injuries and those of an ambulatory nature | Minor fractures and wounds, minor burns of less than 10% body surface area and no respiratory involvement, psychological problems |
| Patients with absence of vital signs | Casualties that have expired or those with injuries that are obviously incompatible with survival |

## APPENDIX A
## Treatment of Airway Problems in Patients with Facial Injuries

| Problem | Treatment |
|---|---|
| **FRACTURE** | |
| Maxilla | Avoid use of nasopharyngeal airway |
| Mandible | Chin pull<br>Oropharyngeal airway (if indicated) |
| **OTHER** | |
| Foreign bodies | Finger sweep and suction to clear blood, clots, loose teeth, etc. |
| Bleeding | Direct pressure with finger in mouth and counterpressure on outside of cheek<br>Pressure points—facial and temporal arteries |
| Uncontrolled bleeding | Lateral recumbent position |
| Inadequate ventilations with above measures | Rapid access to advanced airway techniques |

# APPENDIX B

## Inserting an Esophageal Gastric Tube Airway (EGTA)

1. Place the patient in the supine position, with the head in a neutral or slightly flexed position. Grasp the lower jaw between your thumb and index finger and pull the jaw up away from the pharynx.
2. While maintaining this position, insert the tube against the posterior wall of the pharynx and down into the esophagus until the mask comes in contact with the face. If you encounter resistance, remove the tube and attempt to reinsert.
3. Seal the mask against the face and ventilate through the mask while observing for chest excursions.
4. Once you observe the chest rise, auscultate both lung fields and over the epigastrium with your stethoscope to confirm placement. Then inflate the cuff with 35 mL of air and continue ventilation.

### Contraindications

There are some instances in which the EGTA must not be used. They include the following:

- In children under 16 years of age or less than 5 feet tall. The tube is too long for these individuals.
- Persons over 7 feet tall, since the cuff would rest

*Continued on following page*

# APPENDIX D
## Inserting an Oropharyngeal Airway

1. Measure the airway to ensure proper placement.
2. Place the index finger of one hand on the top teeth and the thumb on the lower teeth and apply pressure in opposite directions (see Figure).
3. Insert the device into the mouth with the tip pointing toward the roof of the mouth.
4. Be careful not to push the tongue into the oropharynx, and rotate the device into place just behind the tongue.

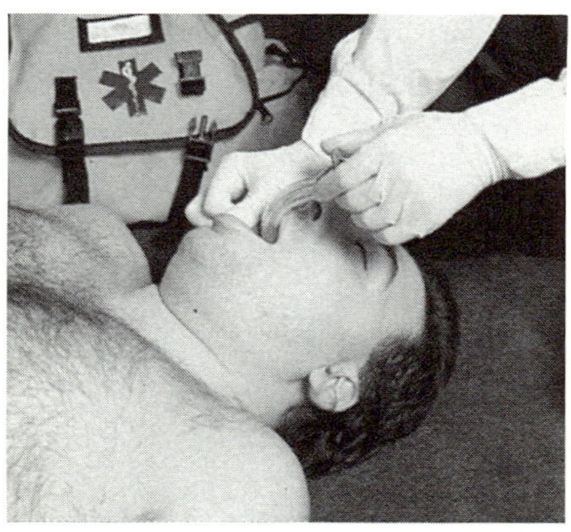

5. *If the patient begins to gag, remove the airway immediately* and do not attempt reinsertion. This could result in vomiting and aspiration of vomitus.
6. Once the airway is in place, test the patency of the airway by ventilating the patient. If you are unable to ventilate, remove the airway, maintain manual maneuvers, and reinsert when possible.

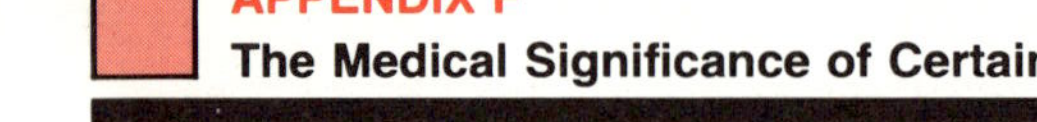

# APPENDIX F

## The Medical Significance of Certain Odors

| Odor | Possible Substance |
|---|---|
| Acetone (sweet, like russet apples) | Ethyl or isopropyl alcohol, chloroform, ketoacidosis, lacquer |
| Acrid (pearlike) | Paraldehyde, chloral hydrate |
| Alcohol (fruitlike) | Ethyl or isopropyl alcohol |
| Ammoniac | Urea |
| Bitter almonds | Cyanide (e.g., in choke cherry or apricot pits) |
| Carrots | Cicutoxin |
| Coal gas (stove gas) | Carbon monoxide (odorless but associated with coal gas) |
| Disinfectants | Phenol, creosote |
| Eggs (rotten) | Hydrogen sulfide, mercaptans, disulfiram (Antabuse) |
| Fecal vomitus | Lower-bowel obstruction |
| Fish or raw liver (musty) | Hepatic failure, zinc phosphorus |
| Fruitlike | Amyl nitrite, ethyl or isopropyl alcohol |

| Odor | Possible Substance |
|---|---|
| Garlic | Phosphorus, tellurium, arsenic (breath and perspiration), parathion, malathion, selenium, dimethyl sulfoxide (DMSO), thallium |
| Gasoline | Kerosene, gasoline |
| Halitosis | Acute illness, poor oral hygiene |
| Mothballs | Camphor-containing products |
| Peanuts | RH-787 (Vacor) |
| Shoe polish | Nitrobenzene |
| Tobacco (stale) | Nicotine |
| Urine | Kidney failure |
| Violets | Urinary turpentine |
| Wintergreen | Methyl salicylate |

Modified from Goldfrank LR: Toxicologic Emergencies, 2nd ed. New York: Appleton-Century-Crofts, 1982, p. 253.

# APPENDIX G

## Management of Drug Overdose and Poisoning

| Drug/Substance | Trade or Street Name |
|---|---|
| **HOUSEHOLD PRODUCTS** | |
| Acids | Toilet bowl cleaners<br>Rust removers<br>Metal cleaners and polishes<br>Tile and grout cleaners |
| Alkalis | Automatic dishwasher detergent<br>Drain cleaners<br>Oven cleaners<br>Washing soda<br>Ammonia<br>Bleach |

| Signs/Symptoms | EMT Management |
|---|---|
| Severe pain in mouth, stomach, chest (substernal) | NEVER INDUCE VOMITING<br>Give patient<br>Milk<br>Milk of magnesia<br>Egg whites (dilutes the acid)<br>Have patient sit up during transport |
| Severe pains in mouth, stomach, chest (substernal)<br>Burns in mouth and esophagus<br>Associated difficulty with swallowing | NEVER INDUCE VOMITING<br>Give milk or water<br>Have patient sit up during transport<br>Watch airway closely for edema causing restricted ventilation |

*Continued on following page*

## APPENDIX G *Continued*

| Drug/Substance | Trade or Street Name |
|---|---|
| Hydrocarbons | Petroleum products |
| | Gasoline |
| | Fuel oils |
| | Paint thinners |
| | Paint solvents |
| | Kerosene |
| | Lighter fluid |
| | Furniture polish |
| Cyanide | Laetrile overdose |
| | Contaminated fruit |
| | Seed crop fumigants |
| | Photochemicals |
| | Electroplating |

| Signs/Symptoms | EMT Management |
|---|---|
| Most common symptoms are respiratory distress with coughing and choking<br>Patient may develop pulmonary edema<br>Abdominal pain may be present<br>Convulsions (seizures)<br>Patient may be comatose<br>Monitor for arrhythmias | NEVER INDUCE VOMITING<br>Treat with up to 100% oxygen depending on severity of overdose<br>Control secretions with suction as required<br>Have patient sit up during transport if possible |
| Initial stage<br>Confusion<br>Rapid respirations<br>Later stage<br>Depressed respirations<br>Vomiting<br>Seizure<br>Comatose | Some paramedic programs have cyanide antidote kits available. Support vital signs and respiration. If antidote kit is not available, transport patient to nearest medical facility having antidote |

*Continued on following page*

| Drug/Substance | Trade or Street Name |
| --- | --- |
| Pesticides | Warfarin base: rat killer<br>Strychnine base: rodenticides<br>Arsenic base: insect sprays, ant and roach killers, liquid insect killers, DDT pesticides, organophosphates |
| Perfumes/Deodorizers | Products containing perfumes and deodorizers are too numerous to list here |

| Drug/Substance | Trade or Street Name |
|---|---|
| Warfarin type<br>Severe gastrointestinal symptoms<br>Progressive lethargy/apathy | Warfarin poisoning:<br>Patient must be seen at hospital for blood-clotting problems |
| Strychinine based<br>Acute illness<br>Severe nausea/vomiting<br>Respiratory distress<br>Tonic stiffening | Patients who are conscious with gag reflex can be given ipecac<br>Support ventilation as required<br>Tonic stiffening requires antiseizure medicines |
| Arsenic based<br>Acute gastrointestinal symptoms | Illicit drugs, e.g., heroin, are sometimes cut with strychnine |
| DDT<br>Severe gastroenteritis | Some pesticides contain anticholinergic agents |
| Produce severe gastroenteritis<br>Respiratory problems from aerosol products may be present | Give oxygen as required<br>Support vital signs |

*Continued on following page*

## APPENDIX G *Continued*

| Drug/Substance | Trade or Street Name |
|---|---|
| **PLANTS** | |
| Poisonous plants | Glycosides |
| | Foxglove |
| | Azalea |
| | Rhododendrons |
| | Alkaloidal toxins |
| | Hemlock |
| | Nightshade |
| | GI irritants |
| | Philodendron |
| | Deiffenbachia |
| | Holly |

| Signs/Symptoms | EMT Management |
|---|---|
| Glycosides | Support with oxygen as required |
| Nausea/vomiting | Support hypotension as with hypovolemia |
| Hypotension | Use cardiac monitor if available |
| May have bradycardia (heart rate <55 per minute) | Bring plant sample to hospital |
| Alkaloidal toxins | |
| Lethargy, which may progress to seizures and coma | |
| GI irritants | |
| Severe nausea/vomiting | |
| Diarrhea | |
| Hypotension | |

*Continued on following page*

**APPENDIX G** ***Continued***

| Drug/Substance | Trade or Street Name |
| --- | --- |
| Poisonous mushrooms | *Amanita muscaria* |
| Hallucinogenic mushrooms | Psilocybin and psilocin |

| Signs/Symptoms | EMT Management |
|---|---|
| 10–30 minutes after ingestion: severe nausea/vomiting followed rapidly by seizures; death may occur | Support with oxygen as required<br>Support hypotension as with hypovolemia<br>Use cardiac monitor if available |
| Severe mood disturbances<br>Hyperventilation<br>Nausea/vomiting<br>Fever<br>Reduced level of consciousness | Use ipecac if patient has gag reflex and is conscious<br>Calm patient as necessary<br>Support vital signs and ventilation as required<br>Bring plant sample to hospital<br>Onset 15–30 minutes after ingestion lasting up to 4–6 hours |

*Continued on following page*

## APPENDIX G *Continued*

| Drug/Substance | Trade or Street Name |
|---|---|
| **DRUGS, SEDATIVES, HYPNOTICS, TRANQUILIZERS** | |
| ***Barbiturates (Long-Acting)*** | |
| Phenobarbital | Luminal (prescription); barbs, purple hearts, downers, yellow jackets (street) |

| Signs/Symptoms | EMT Management |
| --- | --- |
| Constricted pupils | Consult physician concerning ipecac, as drug may depress patient's gag reflex at the same time ipecac begins to work |
| Respiratory depression to complete arrest | Support ventilations and blood pressure as per hypovolemia |
| Gradual onset of lethargy to coma | Check patient's gag reflex and level of consciousness frequently |
| Hypotension | Use cardiac monitor if available |
| Hypothermia | Most abused drug next to Valium and alcohol |

*Continued on following page*

| Drug/Substance | Trade or Street Name |
|---|---|
| ***Barbiturates (Intermediate-Acting)*** | |
| Amobarbital | Amytal (prescription); blue ice, blue lady, turquoise blue birds (street) |
| Secobarbital | Seconal (prescription); red birds, red devils, downers, laybacks, reds (street) |
| Pentobarbital | Nembutal (prescription); block busters, nemmies, nebbies (street) |
| Pentobarbital/Amobarbital combination | Tuinal (prescription); Christmas tree, rainbows, tootsie (street) |

| Signs/Symptoms | EMT Management |
|---|---|
| | May be used to reduce effect of amphetamines causing mixed overdose<br>Usual dose: 15–30 mg three times per day |
| Faster onset but shorter duration than phenobarbital<br>Level of consciousness from agitated to comatose | Same as phenobarbital |
| | Usual dose: 30 mg 3–4 times per day; 100 mg at bedtime |
| Pupils may be small | |

*Continued on following page*

| Drug/Substance | Trade or Street Name |
| --- | --- |
| ***Other Sedatives*** | |
| Glutethimide | Doriden/CB,D |
| Methaqualone | Quaalude (prescription); super/quads, soapers, roarers, ludes (street) |
| Methaqualone hydrochloride | Parest, Soma |

| Signs/Symptoms | EMT Management |
|---|---|
| Rapid onset of coma (1 hour)<br>Stupor or coma may alternate with alert or hyperactive behavior<br>Pupils may be dilated/fixed<br>Sudden apnea and hypotension may occur | Monitor vital signs and ventilation closely<br>Avoid ipecac because coma may develop rapidly<br>Usual dose: 1 tablespoon at bedtime; repeat after 4 hours |
| Sedative-hypnotic, action similar to that of short-acting barbiturates; coma and respiratory depression most common | Support ABCs as required<br>Abrupt withdrawal can cause serious side effects, including seizure, chills, general behavior change, anxiety<br>If mixed with alcohol, drug can be fatal<br>Usual dose: 400 mg at bedtime |
| Possible hallucinations | |

*Continued on following page*

| Drug/Substance | Trade or Street Name |
|---|---|
| Methyprylon | Noludar |
| Meprobamate | Miltown, Equanil, Mepriam, Saronil, Tranmep, Meprospan |
| Ethchlorvynol | Placidyl |

| Signs/Symptoms | EMT Management |
|---|---|
| Pulmonary edema<br>Diaphoresis<br>Drowsiness, nausea, vomiting | |
| Extreme drowsiness progressing to coma<br>Possible hypotension<br>Possible respiratory arrest | This drug is usually slow to produce severe effects; can use ipecac if given within 15–20 min after ingestion of drug<br>Support ABCs as required<br>Large quantity of alcohol makes overdose possible with smaller dose<br>Usual adult dose: 1200–1600 mg per day in divided doses |
| Onset of coma in 1 hour, which can be prolonged for days | Support vital signs and respiration<br>Be prepared for seizure |

*Continued on following page*

## APPENDIX G *Continued*

| Drug/Substance | Trade or Street Name |
|---|---|
| Diazepam | Valium |
| Lorazepam | Ativan |
| Chlordiazepoxide | Librium |
| Flurazepam | Dalmane |
| Clorazepate | Tranxene |
| Oxazepam | Serax |

| Signs/Symptoms | EMT Management |
|---|---|
| Seizures<br>Depressed ventilation<br>Absence of response to painful stimuli | Avoid ipecac, as drug has rapid action in large quantities<br>Combination of Placidyl and amitriptyline can cause patient to be delirious<br>Usual adult dose: 500–1000 mg |
| Unconsciousness from Valium, Ativan, and Tranxene is rapid (10–30 min)<br>Unconsciousness from Librium, Dalmane, and Serax is slow (hours) | Do not use ipecac with Valium, Ativan, and Tranxene because of rapid action of drugs<br>Valium is the most widely prescribed and abused of all sedatives |
| Initially patient will be sleepy, confused; slurred speech with possible difficulty in controlling motor functions will progress to coma, respiratory depression, and/or respiratory arrest | Support vital signs and respiration as required<br>Alcohol is often used with these drugs; makes even small dose unpredictable<br>Usual adult dose: 2–4 mg per day |

*Continued on following page*

## APPENDIX G *Continued*

| Drug/Substance | Trade or Street Name |
|---|---|
| ***Opiates and Derivatives*** | Numbers in parentheses indicate potency equal to 10 mg of morphine sulfate |
| Opium | Paregoric (25 mL) |
| Opium tincture | Morphine |
| Laudanum | Codeine (60–100 mg) |
| Morphine sulfate Heroin | Heroin (3 mg); junk, scag, horse, smack, dreamer, dope (street) |
| Codeine | Dilaudid (2 mg) |
| Diacetylmorphine | Percodan (50 mg) |
| Hydromorphone | Demerol (80–100 mg) |
| Oxycodone | |
| Meperidine | |

| Signs/Symptoms | EMT Management |
|---|---|
| Pupils are small to pinpoint and are nonreactive | Support vital signs; oxygenate and ventilate as necessary |
| Respiratory arrest is common, also shallow slow respirations | Patient may be talking but not have gag to protect airway |
| Patients are stuporous to comatose but are often arousable to painful stimuli; will return to unconsciousness when stimulus is relaxed | Antidote is naloxone (Narcan), which is usually available from paramedics or most medical facilities |
| Patients may have pulmonary edema and/or atrial fibrillation | These patients may have underlying communicable diseases from poor care of needles and poor living habits |
| Look for fresh injection sites in arms, legs, between fingers and toes, as well as tattoos near large veins to hide needle marks | Treat pulmonary edema as required |
| | Strychnine is often used to "cut" opiates; side effect is seizure and hypothermia |
| | Be alert; patients can be dangerous |

*Continued on following page*

## APPENDIX G *Continued*

| Drug/Substance | Trade or Street Name |
|---|---|
| Percodan | |
| Pentazocine | Talwin |
| Methadone | Dolophine (8 mg) Methadone Amidone |
| Oxycodone and acetaminophen | Percocet |
| Propoxyphene | Darvon |
| Propoxyphene and acetaminophen | Darvocet, Darvocet-N |

| Signs/Symptoms | EMT Management |
|---|---|
| | Do not relax vigilance in presence of patient or friends; stick to medical approach only<br>Have police in attendance |
| | Methadone often used in detoxification of heroin addicts; withdrawal symptoms are slower and less severe |
| Pupils may not be pinpoint<br>Can produce all other effects of opiates<br>Darvocet-N may present with symptoms of hypoglycemia | Same as opiates<br>Can be refined and injected |

*Continued on following page*

| Drug/Substance | Trade or Street Name |
|---|---|
| Etorphine hydrochloride | M99 |
| **STIMULANTS** | |
| Amphetamine | Benzedrine (prescription); benz, bennies, speed, uppers (street) |
| Dextroamphetamine | Dexedrine (prescription); dexies, copilots (street) |
| Methamphetamine | Desoxyn, Methedrine, Obedrin-L (prescription); black beauties (street) |

| Signs/Symptoms | EMT Management |
|---|---|
| Is a thousand times more potent than morphine with sedative and respiratory effects | Same as opiates<br>Used only by veterinarians to immobilize large animals |
| Agitation, flushing, perspiration, tachycardia, hypertension | Decrease sensory stimulation; support vital signs and ventilation as required<br>Barbiturates often used to control "high"; therefore patient may have combined symptoms<br>Usual doses: 5–60 mg per day |
| Patient may be hyperactive, with muscle twitching<br>Anxiety with visual hallucinations may occur<br>Nausea, vomiting, abdominal cramps | Handle patient with caution—may have rapid mood changes<br>May require restraints in best interest of patient |

*Continued on following page*

## APPENDIX G *Continued*

| Drug/Substance | Trade or Street Name |
|---|---|
| Amphetamine and dextroamphetamine | Biphenamine |
| Methylphenidate | Ritalin (prescription); ritlins (street) |
| Phenmetrazine<br>Cocaine | Preludin (prescription); snow, coke, white lady, toot, crack (street) |

| Signs/Symptoms | EMT Management |
|---|---|
| Hyperventilation<br>Moderately dilated pupils | Ipecac should be considered if patient has active gag reflex and is conscious |
| When severe, can lead to seizure and coma | Ritalin used for hyperactive children to reduce hyperactivity; often injected, for street use, causing abscesses on skin and "cotton fever" from cotton ball fibers through which drug was strained for injection<br>Usual dose 10–60 mg per day, divided 2–3 times per day |
| Patient often combative, tachycardia, hypertension | Talk down if disoriented<br>Prepare for seizures<br>Oxygenate |

| Drug/Substance | Trade or Street Name |
|---|---|
| **HALLUCINOGENS, PSYCHEDELICS** | |
| DMT (dimethyltryptamine) | |
| LSD | Acid, cubes, purple haze (street) |
| Mescaline | Mesc, cactus (street) |
| Peyote | |
| Psilocybin | Magic mushrooms (street) |
| Phencyclidine | PCP, animal tranquilizer (prescription); angel dust, peace pill, angel fuzz, supergrass (with marijuana) (street) |

| Signs/Symptoms | EMT Management |
| --- | --- |
| Pupils are large<br>Patient is agitated, hot, flushed, delirious with hallucinations<br>Toxic level of LSD usually lasts 12–24 hours | Talk down; orient to surroundings; decrease stimulation<br>Protect patient from injury to EMT(s) and themselves<br>Support vital signs and ventilation as required<br>Combination of hallucinogen and phenothiazines may cause cardiovascular failure, shock, and death |
| Pupils may be mid-size to large<br>Combative behavior changing to depression<br>Respiratory arrest<br>Effect may last 2–4 days<br>Hallucinations | Same as above<br>This patient can be extremely dangerous; patients have been known to break their own limbs during restraint without acknowledging injury |

*Continued on following page*

## APPENDIX G *Continued*

| Drug/Substance | Trade or Street Name |
|---|---|
| Tetrahydrocannabinol | Marijuana, grass, pot, weed, Colombian gold, Thai sticks, etc. (street) |

| Signs/Symptoms | EMT Management |
| --- | --- |
| | PCP can be easily manufactured outside the lab in large quantity, with varied composition as a result<br>Patient may react differently to same-size dose<br>Is used in many forms |
| Anxiety, agitation, loss of interest<br>Large pupils with "bloodshot" whites of eyes<br>Appears drunk<br>Hyperventilation secondary to surprising extra effect of "good" drug | Observation is usually sufficient<br>Occasional hypotension when used in conjunction with alcohol<br>Treat hyperventilation as usual |

*Continued on following page*

## APPENDIX G *Continued*

| Drug/Substance | Trade or Street Name |
|---|---|
| **PSYCHOTROPIC AGENTS** | |
| Phenothiazines | Thorazine, Promapar, Chlor-PZ |
| Chlorpromazine | |
| Trifluoperazine | Stelazine |
| Thioridazine | Mellaril |
| Prochlorperazine | Compazine |
| Haloperidol | Haldol |
| Perphenazine | Trilafon |

| Signs/Symptoms | EMT Management |
| --- | --- |
| Lethargy, which may progress to coma<br>Orthostatic (postural) hypotension to profound hypotension | Treat hypotension with elevated extremities<br>Support ventilation<br>Monitor cardiac arrhythmias if monitor is available<br>All phenothiazines lower the seizure threshold |
| Pulmonary edema (Mellaril)<br>Cardiac arrhythmias<br>Dystonic reactions (swollen tongue, rigid jaw with face distorted) | Be prepared for cardiac and/or respiratory arrest<br>High-flow oxygen or bag mask assist |
| Limbs tonic, respiratory distress<br>Seizures | These patients require immediate care to treat severe symptoms early<br>Patient can become extremely ill rapidly |

*Continued on following page*

## APPENDIX G *Continued*

| Drug/Substance | Trade or Street Name |
| --- | --- |
| **ANTIDEPRESSANTS** | |
| Tricyclics | |
| Amitriptyline | Elavil, Endep |
| Imipramine | Tofranil |
| Desipramine | Norpramin |
| Nortriptyline | Aventyl |
| Doxepin | Sinequan |
| Amitriptyline and perphenazine | Triavil, Etrafon |
| MAO inhibitors | Parnate |
| | Marplan |
| | Niamid |
| | Nardil |

| Signs/Symptoms | EMT Management |
|---|---|
| Patients are often excited but can progress rapidly to coma<br>Tachycardia and arrhythmias are very common | Treat same as phenothiazines<br>Patient can become extremely ill rapidly<br>Cardiac arhythmias with sudden death are the greatest danger |
| Hypertension or hypotension<br>Seizures<br>May have symptoms of phenothiazines and tricyclics | Foods such as cheese and wine may cause symptoms of toxicity |
| Same as tricyclics | |

*Continued on following page*

## APPENDIX G *Continued*

| Drug/Substance | Trade or Street Name |
|---|---|
| **ATROPINIC ANTICHOLINERGICS** | |
| Belladonna | Atropine, belladonna |
| **ANTIHISTAMINES** | |
| Diphenhydramine | Benadryl |
| Dimenhydrinate | Dramamine |

| Signs/Symptoms | EMT Management |
|---|---|
| Classic atropine intoxication<br>Delirious ("mad as a hatter"), flushed ("red as a beet"), dilated pupils ("blind as a bat"), absent perspiration ("dry as a bone") | Control hypotension as required<br>Control hyperthermia as required<br>Jimson weed and nightshade contain belladonna |
| Sedative effect with low dosage | Same as anticholinergics<br>Commonly used by public as antinausea medicine |
| Symptoms the same as anticholinergics in high dosage | |

*Continued on following page*

## APPENDIX G *Continued*

| Drug/Substance | Trade or Street Name |
|---|---|
| **MILD ANALGESICS** | |
| Salicylate | Aspirin and others (over 400 preparations contain salicylate) |
| Acetaminophen | Tylenol, Datril, often combined with mild opiates |
| **OTHER COMPOUNDS** | |
| Phenytoin | Dilantin |

| Signs/Symptoms | EMT Management |
|---|---|
| Initial symptoms: headache, nausea, hyperventilation<br>Later symptoms: lethargy to coma<br>Seizures<br>Increased perspiration, hyperthermia | Use ipecac as soon as possible if patient is conscious; aspirin tends to form hard "ball" in stomach if not removed. |
| Nausea, general ill feeling<br>Liver damage may occur in large quantity overdoses after 24 hours | Use ipecac as soon as possible if patient is conscious<br>Administer large quantities of fluid orally to cause excretion naturally |
| Slurred speech, hypotension | Support vital signs and ventilation |

*Continued on following page*

**APPENDIX G** ***Continued***

| Drug/Substance | Trade or Street Name |
| --- | --- |
| Lithium | Eskalith<br>Lithane |

| Signs/Symptoms | EMT Management |
|---|---|
| Occasional dystonic posturing (see phenothiazine)<br>Coma is rare except with massive overdose<br>May develop AV block arrhythmia | Cardiac monitor if available; be prepared to assist heart block with CPR should hypotension occur<br>Overdose may be accidental, as each patient's ability to metabolize this drug varies |
| Muscle tremor, blackout spells, slurred speech, dizziness, blurred vision, dry mouth, fatigue, lethargy, confusion, stupor, coma; early signs of diarrhea, vomiting, dizziness | Support vital signs and ventilation<br>Lithium toxicity is closely related to serum lithium levels, and can occur at doses close to therapeutic levels<br>Treats manic-depressive patients only |

*Continued on following page*

## APPENDIX G *Continued*

| Drug/Substance | Trade or Street Name |
|---|---|
| Iron | |
| Ferrous gluconate | Fergon |
| Ferrous sulfate | Feosol, Mol-Iron, others |
| Ferrous fumarate | Feostat, others |
| **ALCOHOL COMPOUNDS** | |
| Ethanol | "Alcohol" |

| Signs/Symptoms | EMT Management |
|---|---|
| Nausea, vomiting, diarrhea, stomach upset, weak/rapid pulse, decreased blood pressure | Induce vomiting with ipecac<br>Hospital must pump stomach within first hour, as stomach may perforate from treatment |
| Heavy dose can cause brisk bleeding in stomach/intestine and black tarry stools (from hemorrhage)<br>Shock | |
| "Drunkenness"-like symptoms, coma, and respiratory depression with large quantities | Normally supportive |

*Continued on following page*

## APPENDIX G *Continued*

| Drug/Substance | Trade or Street Name |
|---|---|
| Methanol | Sterno |
| Ethylene glycol | Antifreeze |

Modified from Copass MK, Soper RG, Eisenberg S: EMT Manual, 2nd ed. Philadelphia: WB Saunders, 1991.

| Signs/Symptoms | EMT Management |
| --- | --- |
| Loss of gag reflex<br>Dilated, slow-reacting pupils | May require aggressive airway management with children and young adults (often first-time users)<br>Often used mixed with a variety of drugs |
| Usually takes 8–36 hours to take effect: headache, blurred vision, seizures, nausea, vomiting, abdominal cramps, to coma | Main treatment is performed by hospital<br>Contact physician for ipecac in field<br>As little as 2 teaspoons can be toxic; 2–8 oz can be fatal |
| Hyperventilation<br>Coma occurs rapidly; may cause pulmonary edema seizures | Same as methanol<br>As little as 100 mL may cause coma |

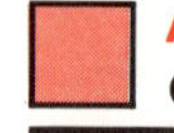

# APPENDIX H
## Other Commonly Abused Substances

| Drug | Street Name |
|---|---|
| Alcohol | Booze, brew, hooch |
| Nicotine | Smoke, butt, coffin nail |
| Airplane glue*<br>Paint thinner* | |

| Symptoms and Signs | EMT Management |
|---|---|
| Impaired coordination | Treat symptomatically |
| Impaired judgment | Talk down if disoriented |
| | If unconscious, oxygenate and place on side |
| Tobacco smell | If swallowed, keep on side for vomiting |
| Stained teeth | |
| Poor motor coordination | High-flow oxygen and assist |
| Impaired vision | ↓ Sensory stimulation |
| Violent behavior | |

*Continued on following page*

## APPENDIX H *Continued*

| Drug | Street Name |
|---|---|
| Nitrous oxide | Laughing gas, whippets |
| Amyl nitrite | Poppers, rush, locker room, snappers, amies |

*The active agent in airplane glue and paint thinner is toluene. Naphtha, methyl ethyl ketone, and gasoline may produce similar symptoms.

Modified from the Department of Transportation Emergency Medical Technician National Standard Curriculum, 1985.

| Symptoms and Signs | EMT Management |
|---|---|
| Hilarity | Talk down |
| Euphoria | Oxygenate |
| Lightheadedness | |
| Hilarity | Talk down if necessary |
| Dizziness | Oxygenate |
| Headache | |
| Impaired thought | |

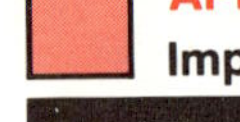

# APPENDIX I
## Important Phone Numbers

HAZ-MAT Incidents (including radiation accidents):
 Chemtrex (800) 424-9300 (24-hour service)

Radiation Accidents:
 Radiation Emergency Assistance Center/Training Site (REACT/TS):
  (615) 576-3131 (Monday through Friday 8:00 A.M. to 4:30 P.M.)
  (615) 481-1000, beeper 241 (24-hour service at Oak Ridge Hospital)

Poison Control Center:

______________________________

Other important phone numbers:

______________________________

______________________________

______________________________

______________________________

______________________________

# APPENDIX J

## Adult Trauma Score

| | Coded Value |
|---|---|
| **SYSTOLIC BLOOD PRESSURE** | |
| >89 | 4 |
| 76–89 | 3 |
| 50–75 | 2 |
| 1–49 | 1 |
| 0 | 0 |
| **RESPIRATORY RATE** | |
| 10–29 | 4 |
| >29 | 3 |
| 6–9 | 2 |
| 1–5 | 1 |
| 0 | 0 |
| **GLASGOW COMA SCALE** | |
| 13–15 | 4 |
| 9–12 | 3 |
| 6–8 | 2 |
| 4–5 | 1 |
| 3 | 0 |
| SCORE | 0 to 12 |
| Scoring triage criterion for direct transport of the patient to a trauma center | ≤11 |

Trauma scoring standardizes the description of injury severity. Trauma scoring is an essential step in the management of trauma patients for appropriate triage, hospital transfer, and assurance of quality of care.

From American College of Surgeons Committee on Trauma 1988.

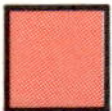

## APPENDIX K
## Pediatric Trauma Score

| | Coded Value |
|---|---|
| **SIZE** | |
| >20 kg | +2 |
| 10–20 kg | +1 |
| <10 kg | −1 |
| **AIRWAY** | |
| Normal | +2 |
| Maintainable | +1 |
| Not maintainable | −1 |
| **SYSTOLIC BLOOD PRESSURE (BP)** | |
| >90 mm Hg | +2 |
| 50–90 mm Hg | +1 |
| <50 mm Hg | −1 |
| *In the absence of proper size BP cuff, assess BP by assigning these values:* | |
| Pulse palpable at wrist | +2 |
| Pulse palpable at groin | +1 |
| Pulse not palpable | −1 |
| **CENTRAL NERVOUS SYSTEM STATUS** | |
| Awake | +2 |
| Partially conscious or unconscious | +1 |
| Comatose or decerebrate | −1 |

| | |
|---|---|
| **OPEN WOUNDS** | |
| None | +2 |
| Minor | +1 |
| Major | −1 |
| **SKELETAL INJURY** | |
| None | +2 |
| Closed fracture | +1 |
| Open/multiple fractures | −1 |
| SCORE | −6 to +12 |
| Scoring triage criterion for direct transport of the patient to a trauma center | <9 |

From American College of Surgeons Committee on Trauma 1988.

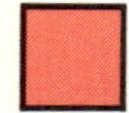

## APPENDIX L
## Pediatric Glasgow Coma Scale

| Category | Response | Score |
|---|---|---|
| Verbal | Coos, babbles, or cries spontaneously | 5 |
| | Irritable crying | 4 |
| | Cries to pain | 3 |
| | Moans to pain | 2 |
| | None | 1 |
| Motor | Spontaneous movement | 6 |
| | Withdraws to touch | 5 |
| | Withdraws to pain | 4 |
| | Abnormal flexion | 3 |
| | Abnormal extension | 2 |
| | None | 1 |
| Eye opening | Spontaneous | 4 |
| | To speech | 3 |
| | To pain | 2 |
| | None | 1 |

Adapted from James, H.E. Neurologic evaluation and support in the child with acute brain insult. *Pediatric Annals* 15(1):17, 1986.

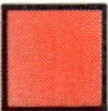

## APPENDIX M
## Medical Abbreviations *Continued*

**EMT:** Emergency medical technician
**ET:** Endotracheal
**ETA:** Estimated time of arrival
**ETOH:** Ethyl alcohol
**Fx:** Fracture
**GI:** Gastrointestinal
**g** (or **gm**): Gram
**GSW:** Gunshot wound
**gtt:** Drops
**Gyn:** Gynecologic
**H&P:** History and physical
**HR:** Heart rate
**Hx:** History
**ICU:** Intensive care unit
**IM:** Intramuscular
**IUD:** Intrauterine device
**IV:** Intravenous
**Kg:** Kilogram
**LLQ:** Left lower quadrant
**L/m:** Liters per minute
**LMP:** Last menstrual period
**LOC:** Level of consciousness
**LS:** Lung sounds
**LUQ:** Left upper quadrant
**MAST:** Military antishock trousers (same as PASG)
**mcg** or **μg:** Microgram
**MI:** Myocardial infarction
**mL:** Milliliter
**mm:** Millimeter
**MOI:** Mechanism of injury

## APPENDIX M
### Medical Abbreviations *Continued*

**MVA:** Motor vehicle accident
**NaCl:** Sodium chloride
**$NaHCO_3$:** Sodium bicarbonate
**NG:** Nasogastric
**NS:** Normal saline
**NSR:** Normal sinus rhythm
**$O_2$:** Oxygen
**OB:** Obstetrics
**OD:** Overdose
**OR:** Operating room
**PASG:** Pneumatic antishock garment (same as MAST)
**PDR:** *Physicians' Desk Reference*
**PE:** Physical examination
**PH:** Past history
**PI:** Present illness
**PO:** By mouth
**PRN:** As necessary
**Pt:** Patient
**q̄:** Every
**q̄d:** Every day
**q̄h:** Every hour
**qid:** Four times a day
**RLQ:** Right lower quadrant
**RUQ:** Right upper quadrant
**Rx:** Prescription
**s̄:** Without
**SIDS:** Sudden infant death syndrome

*Continued on following page*

## APPENDIX M
## Medical Abbreviations *Continued*

**SQ:** Subcutaneous
**Stat:** Immediately
**STD:** Sexually transmitted disease
**T:** Temperature
**tid:** Three times a day
**TKO:** To keep open
**TPR:** Temperature, pulse, and respiration
**Tx:** Treatment or traction
**VS:** Vital signs
**w/:** With
**WD:** Well developed
**w/o:** Without
**y.o.:** Year old

# APPENDIX N
## Spell Check

**A**

abdomen
abnormal
abort
abortion
abrasion
abruptio
abscess
absorption
accident
ache
acute
addiction
adhesive
adolescent
advanced
advice
advised
aerosol
agonal
airway
alcohol
alcoholic
allergy
Alzheimer's
ambulatory
amnesia
amniotic
amputation
anaphylactic
anaphylaxis
anemia
aneurysm
angina
ankle
anorexia
anoxia
antecubital
anxiety
APGAR
aphasia
apnea/apneic
appendectomy
appendicitis
appetite
arteriosclerosis
arthritis
artificial
asphyxiate
asphyxiated
asphyxiation
aspirate
aspiration
aspirin
asthma
asthmatic
asystole
aura
auscultate
auscultation
avulsion

*Continued on following page*

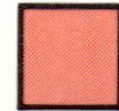

# APPENDIX N
## Spell Check *Continued*

### B

bacteria
balance
bandage
battered
Battle's sign
bedsore
behavior
benign
bilateral
biopsy
birth
bleeding
blind
blinking
blood
boil
bolus
botulism
brady
brain
breath
breathe
breathing
breech
bridge
bronchiolitis
bronchitis
bronchospasm
bulimia
bypass

### C

calcification
cancer
cannula
capsule
carcinoma
cardiac
cardiogenic
cardioversion
carpal-tunnel
carpopedal
castration
casualty
cataract
catatonic
catheter
catheterize
caustic
cavity
central
cerebral
cerebrovascular
cervical
cesarean
chancre
chemotherapy
Cheyne-Stokes
chickenpox
childbirth
chiropractic
chiropractor

chlamydia
cholesterol
chronic
cirrhosis
clavical
clinical
clotting
collapse
colostomy
comatose
compensation
compensatory
complaint
complication
compound
compress
concussion
condition
confused
congenital
congestion
congestive
conscious
consent
constipation
constrict
constriction
contagious
contraction
contraindication
confused
confusion
convalescent
coroner
coughing
counselor
cradle
cramp
cravat
crepitus
critical
croup
crowning
cyanosis
cyanotic
cystic fibrosis

**D**

daughter
deaf
deafness
debridement
decapitate
decapitation
decerebrate
decompression
decorticate
defecate
defibrillate
defibrillation
deformity
degenerative
dehydration
delirium
delivery
delusion
dementia
denial
denture
dependence

*Continued on following page*

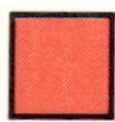

## APPENDIX N
## Spell Check *Continued*

depression
depressive
detached
deviated
diabetes
diabetic
dialysis
diaphoresis
diaphoretic
diaphragm
diarrhea
diastolic
digestion
dilation
diminished
disability
disabled
discharge
disease
dislocation
disoriented
dispatch
dissect
dissection
distal
distension
dizziness
doll's eyes
dosage
Down's syndrome
drainage
dwarfism
dying
dysentery
dysfunction
dyslexia
dyspnea
dystrophy

### E

earache
eardrum
ecchymosis
eclampsia
ectopic
edema
electrocuted
electrode
electrolyte
elimination
embedded
embolism
emergency
emesis
emphysema
endotracheal
enlarge
epiglottitis
epilepsy
epileptic
epistaxis
esophageal
evisceration
examination
excretion
exhale
exhalation
exhaust

exhaustion
expiratory
explosion
exposure
extension
external
extrication
extubate

**F**

fatal
fatality
fatigue
febrile
feces
femur
fetus
fever
fibrillation
flaccid
flail
flea
flush
flutter
forceps
forearm
forehead
fracture
frostbite
fungus

**G**

gag
gallstone
gangrene
gauge
geriatrics
gestation
glaucoma
glucose
gonorrhea
grand mal
gynecology

**H**

hallucination
headache
heat
Heimlich
hematemesis
hematoma
hemodialysis
hemophilia
hemorrhage
hemorrhagic
hepatitis
hernia
herpes
hiatal
hiccup
history
hives
Hodgkin's
homicide
hospice
hyper/hypo
hyperactive
hyperthermia
hyperventilate
hypothermia

*Continued on following page*

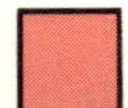

# APPENDIX N
## Spell Check *Continued*

hypovolemia
hypovolemic
hypoxia
hypoxic
hysterectomy
hysterical

**I**

identify
identification
immediate
immobilize
immunity
impairment
impaled
implant
incidence
incident
incision
include
including
incontinent
increase
indentation
indication
indigestion
induce
industrial
infant
infarction
infection
inflammation
infusion
ingestion
inhalation
injection
inspiration
insulin
insurance
intentional
intermittent
intoxication
intraosseous
intravenous
intubation
involuntary
irrational
irregular
irritate
irritation
ischemia

**J**

jaundice
joule
jugular

**K**

ketoacidosis
kidney
Kussmaul

**L**

laceration
lactation
laryngospasm
larynx
lateral

lavage
lesion
lethargy
leukemia
lice
liver
lividity
localized
lower
lymph
lymphatic

**M**

malaria
malignancy
malignant
mania/manic
manipulation
mastectomy
maternal
measles
mechanism
medic
Medicaid
Medicare
medication
medicine
memory
meningitis
menopause
menstrual
mental
mentally
metabolize
migraine
miscarriage
mobility
mononucleosis
mottled
mucous
multiple sclerosis
muscular dystrophy
myocardial

**N**

narcolepsy
nasal
nausea
nebulizer
necrosis
necrotic
needle
neonate
neonatal
neurogenic
neurological
nose/nostril
nurse
nursing

**O**

obese
obey
obstetrician
obstructed
obstruction
occlude
occluded
organic
orientation

*Continued on following page*

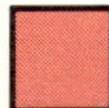

# APPENDIX N
## Spell Check *Continued*

oropharyngeal
orthopneic
osteoporosis
outpatient
overdose
ovulation

**P**

pacemaker
pallor
palpation
palpitation
paradoxical
paralysis
paralyzed
paranoid
paraplegic
parasite
parasitic
Parkinson's
patient
pedestrian
pediatric
pelvis
penis
percussion
perforation
perfusion
pericardial
peripheral
petit mal
phlebitis
phobia
physical
physician
pitting
placenta
pleurisy
pneumonia
pneumothorax
poison
position
postictal
posterior
posture
posturing
preeclampsia
pregnant
premature
prenatal
prescription
presentation
previa
priapism
prolapsed
prosthesis
psychiatric
psychiatrist
psychotic
pubic
pulmonary
pulsating
pulse
puncture

**O**

quadrant
quadriplegic
quarantine

**R**

rabies
raccoon sign
radiation
radical
radiology
rales
rash
reaction
rectum
reflex
regulated
relief
remission
resistance
respiration
respiratory
response
restrained
resuscitate
retardation
retention
retraction
rheumatic
rheumatoid
rhonchi
rhythm
rigidity
rigor mortis
rotation
rupture

**S**

saliva
sanitary
scalp
schizophrenia
scorpion
scrotum
secondary
seizure
sensation
sensitive
septic
shock
shunt
sickle cell
sinus
skull
sneeze
snoring
spasm
splint
spontaneous
sprain
sputum
status
sternum
stethoscope
stillbirth
stoma
stool
strain

*Continued on following page*

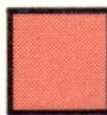

# APPENDIX N
## Spell Check *Continued*

stridor
stroke
stupor
stylet
subdural
sublingual
suction
suffocate
suicide
superficial
supine
suppository
surgery
suture
swallowing
sympathetic
symptom
symptomatic
syncope
syndrome
syphilis
syringe
systolic

### T

tachycardia
tachypnea
tamponade
tearing
technician
teeth
temperature
tender
tenderness
tendon
tension
terminal
testicle
tetanus
therapy
thermometer
thirst
thorax
thready
throbbing
thrombosis
tonic-clonic
topical
tourniquet
toxemia
trachea
tracheal
tracheostomy
traction
transfusion
trauma
traumatic
traumatized
Trendelenburg
triage
triangular
trichinosis
trimester
tuberculosis
tumor

**U**

ulcer
umbilical
unconscious
urine
urinary

**V**

vagina
vasoconstriction
vasodilation
vein
venereal
venom
ventilation
ventricular
vertebra
vertigo
viable
viral
virus
visual
voluntary
vomit
vomitus

**W**

wheeze
withdrawal
wrist

# INDEX

Note: Page numbers in italics refer to illustrations; page numbers followed by t refer to tables.

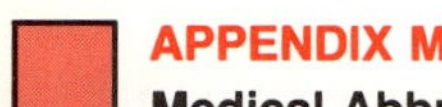

# APPENDIX M
## Medical Abbreviations

**AIDS:** Acquired immunodeficiency syndrome
**ASAP:** As soon as possible
**AX:** Axillary
**BM:** Bowel movement
**BP:** Blood pressure
**BSA:** Body surface area
**BVM:** Bag-valve-mask
**c̄:** With
**CA:** Cancer
**CAD:** Coronary artery disease
**CC:** Chief complaint
**CCU:** Cardiac care unit
**CHF:** Congestive heart failure
**CNS:** Central nervous system
**C/O:** Complains of
**COPD:** Chronic obstructive pulmonary disease
**CP:** Chest pain
**CPR:** Cardiopulmonary resuscitation
**CSF:** Cerebrospinal fluid
**CVA:** Cerebrovascular accident
**DC:** Discontinue
**DOA:** Dead on arrival
**DT:** Delirium tremens
**DV:** Demand valve
**Dx:** Diagnosis
**ECG** (or **EKG**): Electrocardiogram
**ED** (or **ER**): Emergency department (or room)
**EMS:** Emergency medical services

*Continued on following page*